HOW DO I ANSWER THAT?

A SECONDARY SCHOOL TEACHER'S GUIDE TO ANSWERING RSE QUESTIONS

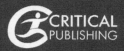

HOW DO I ANSWER THAT?

A SECONDARY SCHOOL TEACHER'S GUIDE TO ANSWERING RSE QUESTIONS

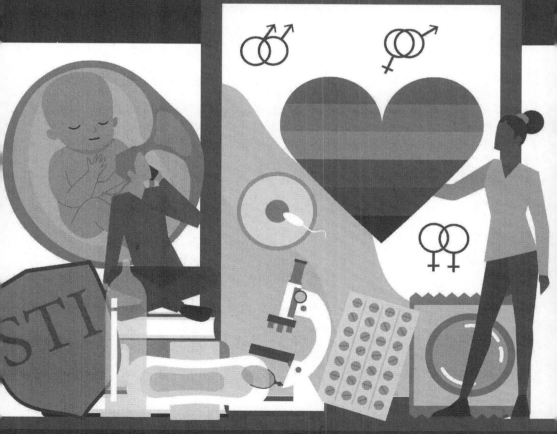

Rachel Scales

First published in 2021 by Critical Publishing Ltd

British Library Cataloguing in Publication Data
A CIP record for this book is available from the British Library

ISBN: 978-1-913453-77-0

This book is also available in the following e-book formats:

EPUB ISBN: 978-1-913453-79-4
Adobe e-book ISBN: 978-1-913453-80-0

Cover and text design by Out of House Limited
Project management by Newgen Publishing UK
Printed and bound in Great Britain by 4edge, Essex

Critical Publishing
3 Connaught Road
St Albans
AL3 5RX

www.criticalpublishing.com

Paper from responsible sources

✚ CONTENTS

✚ MEET THE AUTHOR

RACHEL SCALES

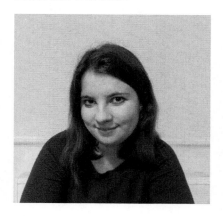 I have been a relationships and sex education (RSE) coordinator and am currently a teacher working at a secondary school in Essex. I have taught RSE in over 20 different schools across London and Essex to thousands of students. I know how daunting it can be to teach RSE, especially when a student asks a question you do not know how to answer. How do you strike the balance between an answer that is professional but open, that is correct but does not scare your pupil? To save you time, I have created this handy and accessible RSE resource to build your confidence and provide pre-prepared, up-to-date, factual answers to the questions students often ask during RSE.

AUTHOR'S NOTE

While I have used the words 'men', 'women', 'girls' and 'boys' in this book, it is always important to consider that not all pupils identify within the stereotypical gender binary. In order to be inclusive, it is important to explore with pupils what these words connotate and if they may be uncomfortable for some pupils.

✚ ACKNOWLEDGEMENTS

This book would not have been possible without the support and encouragement of so many people. I would like to thank Julia Morris at Critical Publishing for seeing the potential in this book and bringing it to print as well as her fantastic support during the process of writing this book.

My thanks go to the many schools and colleges that allowed me to teach RSE to their wonderful pupils and to Brook for shaping me into an open and knowledgeable sex educator.

I would like to thank my friends for their continued support; in particular, Rachel Gambling for helping me conceptualise this book in its early stages; Rebecca Tye and Leona Chapman for their critiques and reads of my draft chapters; Mollie Pye for her constant unwavering support and Shaw Rayment for always believing in my ability to write.

My Dad, Mark, for proofreading chapters and helping me with the photography exhibited in this book. My Mum, Ruth, for always being my number one fan and being my first and favourite RSE teacher. My amazing brother Joshua, who helped contribute to many of the questions in this book and for being proud, never embarrassed, by the fact that his big sister is a sex educator.

Finally, to my partner Josh, thank you for all your love, support and encouragement during the writing of this book. But most importantly, thank you for your excellent tea-making skills. The one thing that stunts writing is a bad cup of tea and thanks to you, I never had to experience this. You are my all-time favourite.

✚ INTRODUCTION

WHY IS RSE NEEDED?

Relationships and sex education (RSE) is a necessity. Not only is it a necessity but unlike other more academic subjects on the secondary school curriculum, RSE has the potential to improve pupils' lives and their relationships going forward. On a grander scale, RSE has the potential to instigate positive societal change: improving tolerance, deepening understanding of consent and improving public health.

HOW OFTEN SHOULD YOU TEACH RSE?

The guidance provided by the Department for Education does not stipulate how often a secondary school is required to teach RSE. Therefore, it is the decision of individual schools to plan how often RSE should be taught. It is good practice that all pupils in secondary school receive RSE at least once during every academic year. This could be delivered as part of a special personal, social, health and economic education (PSHE)/RSE day where pupils are off their usual academic timetable. Other ways RSE can be delivered is through a regular timetabled lesson that occasionally takes the place of a PSHE, citizenship or well-being lesson. RSE can also be delivered during form time and through year group assemblies. Certain RSE topics that are interdisciplinary can also be taught during science and religious studies lessons. For example, discussing the menstrual cycle as part of biology in science or exploring different views on abortion during religious studies.

WHICH TOPICS DO YOU HAVE TO TEACH?

The guidance set out by the Department for Education details what pupils should be expected to know by the end of their secondary school education. It splits the RSE curriculum into five main categories.

1

1. **Families**

   The different types of stable relationships, legal aspects of marriage and the responsibilities parents have towards children.

2. **Respectful relationships, including friendships**

   Factors that make a relationship/friendship healthy or unhealthy, understanding criminal relationships and coercion, the different types of bullying including cyber bullying, good communication and managing conflict within a relationship/friendship.

3. **Online and media**

   Staying safe when sharing personal information online, the impact and risks of pornography, the impact and risks of sharing and viewing indecent images of a child, online privacy and security.

4. **Being safe**

   Understanding sexual and non-sexual consent within relationships; being aware of issues where consent is not given such as rape, sexual assault, female genital mutilation (FGM) and forced marriage; being aware of grooming, honour-based violence and domestic violence.

5. **Intimate and sexual relationships including sexual health**

   Strategies for identifying and managing sexual pressure, information about sexually transmitted infections (STIs), contraception, pregnancy, abortion and how drugs and alcohol can impact decisions in sexual scenarios.

In addition to the above categories, pupils should be expected to know the current laws around the following topics:

+ *marriage;*

+ *consent, including the age of consent;*

+ *violence against women and girls;*

+ *online behaviours including image and information sharing (including 'sexting', youth-produced sexual imagery, nudes, etc)*

+ *pornography;*

+ *abortion;*

+ *sexuality;*

+ *gender identity;*

+ *substance misuse;*

+ *violence and exploitation by gangs;*

+ *extremism and radicalisation;*

+ *criminal exploitation (for example, through gang involvement or 'county lines' drugs operations);*

+ *hate crime;*

+ *female genital mutilation (FGM).*

(DfE, 2019)

PARENTAL WITHDRAWAL FROM RSE

According to the guidance on delivering RSE (DfE, 2019), parents have the right to withdraw their child from any lessons that contain 'sex education'. This right stands until three terms before their child turns 16. For most pupils this will be at some point during Year 10. If a child later wants to receive sex education the school should consider the pupil's wishes. In secondary school, a child cannot be withdrawn from any lessons that cover 'relationships education' or 'health education'. Schools may struggle to differentiate what should be considered 'sex education' and what should be considered as 'relationships education' and 'health education'. Many topics in RSE do overlap and could be considered as 'relationship', 'sex' or 'health' education (see Table 0.1) but as a general rule topics that deal with the more social side of 'sex education' are the ones that pupils would be withdrawn from.

It is also good practice that if some pupils have missed previous RSE lessons due to parental withdrawal then during Year 10 the school should facilitate an RSE catch-up programme for those pupils so they do not completely miss out on vital RSE knowledge.

TABLE 0.1 A breakdown of RSE topics by relationship, health and sex education

Relationship education topics (cannot be withdrawn)	Health education topics (cannot be withdrawn)	Sex education topics (can be withdrawn upon request)
Healthy and unhealthy relationships	Puberty	Contraception
Safe online friendships	Menstrual cycle and period poverty	STIs
Consent and healthy boundaries in relationships	Reproduction and the stages of pregnancy	Sexual pleasure
Communication	Infertility and miscarriage	Pornography
Lesbian, gay, bisexual, transgender and questioning plus all other sexualities (LGBTQ+) relationships and equality	FGM	Sexting

IS RSE OFSTED INSPECTED?

From the summer term of 2021, schools will have been expected to have implemented a comprehensive RSE curriculum. Due to the new mandatory status of RSE within the secondary school curriculum, key aspects of relationships education, RSE and health education are in scope for Ofsted inspection (DfE, 2019). This means Ofsted inspectors could possibly ask to see a copy of your school's RSE curriculum, ask staff when and how often RSE is delivered and ask pupils when they last received RSE. Even though RSE is not an academic subject, Ofsted inspectors may ask to see evidence of pupils' work in RSE.

SKILLS NEEDED TO BE A SUCCESSFUL RSE TEACHER

The most important skills an RSE teacher needs are openness, a non-judgemental attitude and knowledge. By being open and honest about RSE topics you will immediately be presenting to pupils that RSE is not only important but also not a taboo subject. If you are uncomfortable with the topics you are teaching this will make pupils also feel uncomfortable. Effective RSE cannot take place when both staff and pupils are uncomfortable as this classroom atmosphere makes it more likely for teachers to rush through content and not cover it in enough detail. It will also make pupils less likely to ask the questions they want to ask about topics.

A non-judgemental attitude is also imperative to being a successful RSE teacher. While teaching RSE, pupils may disclose information or views to you that you personally don't agree with. A classic example is pupils engaging in sexual activity while they are underage. Though this may be difficult to hear, it is important to remember that you are not there to judge pupils on their sexual behaviours but to give them knowledge so they can make informed choices about their sexual health and relationships. Your facial expressions and body language are key in reflecting a non-judgemental attitude. A shocked reaction from a teacher can be enough to discourage a pupil from ever seeking help or asking a question again. It is vital then that if a pupil asks you a question that you find shocking or don't personally agree with, you should maintain a neutral facial expression and open body language; for example, don't stand with your hands on your hips, crossed arms or put your head in your hands in despair.

EXAMPLE

14 year-old pupil: *Is it true you don't have to use contraception if you have sex standing up? I heard you don't get pregnant or STIs if you have sex standing up.*

This may be perceived as quite a shocking question by most teachers. It is important not to jump to any assumptions just from one question. Just because pupils have asked a question like this, it does not mean they are engaging in unsafe sexual activity. Most knowledge pupils have about sex and sexual health comes from information from friends and social media. It is not uncommon for this information to be incorrect and pupils to be misinformed. Due to the misinformation and myths around sex and relationships, pupils' questions like the one above are more common than one might think. If you need time to consider an answer to a pupil's question, it is always a good technique to ground and thank the pupil for asking the question.

5

EXAMPLE

Teacher's response: *That is a really interesting question; thank you for asking that as I'm sure other pupils were also wondering if that's true. This is a common myth around pregnancies and STIs. When you say 'sex standing up' do you mean vaginal sex? Different sexual positions do not decrease the risk of STIs or an unwanted pregnancy. This means there is still a risk of STIs and unwanted pregnancy if you have vaginal sex standing up. The only thing that will decrease your risk of STIs and unwanted pregnancies is if you use contraception such as a condom during sex.*

This is an excellent response from the teacher as it first reassures the pupil that the question was not silly or stupid. It also clarifies what type of sex the pupil was referring to. Pupils will rarely specify a sexual activity by saying 'vaginal sex', 'anal sex' or 'sexual touching'. So, it's important that you clarify what type of sex they are referring to. Finally, this response gives practical information about the risks of engaging in sexual activity without using contraception. The way the information is delivered is non-judgemental, concise and does not scaremonger. If a pupil ever asks a question that you feel concerned about, it is always a best practice to follow your school's safeguarding policy and have a conversation with a senior member of staff responsible for safeguarding.

Knowledge is the final skill that any successful RSE teacher needs. Just because RSE is not an academic subject, it should not be dismissed as an 'easy' subject to teach. Like academic subjects, it is comprised of many different topic areas. Yet, unlike academic subjects, if a teacher were to give incorrect information during RSE this could have very serious real-world consequences for pupils. To avoid this, teachers responsible for delivering RSE need to be regularly trained in RSE as part of continued professional development (CPD). There are many charities such as Brook, Terrance Higgins Trust and The Sex Education Forum that offer training on RSE topics. It is also worth researching what training is available from your local sexual health provider/local authority. If a pupil asks you a question that you don't know the answer to, it is always better to admit that you don't know the answer rather than give an answer that might not be correct. This is how misinformation is easily spread. You can also direct pupils to different reliable sources that may have the answer to their questions (please see the 'Sources of further information' section at the end of each chapter).

BUILDING AN INCLUSIVE AND OPEN ATMOSPHERE WITHIN THE CLASSROOM

A classroom where pupils feel safe and included is vital to teaching RSE effectively. As the educator, it is your responsibility to set the tone for how you expect pupils to behave not just towards you but towards each other during an RSE lesson. You will receive a mixed reaction from pupils at the beginning of an RSE lesson. Depending on the topic, pupils could show shock, embarrassment, curiosity, interest, rebelliousness or mocking behaviour. Due to these emotions and the behaviours pupils may exhibit, it is a good idea to set some ground rules or expectations before the lesson starts. These ground rules could be:

+ respecting other classmates by listening to them and not laughing at them;

+ respecting the teacher by not asking personal questions;

+ not telling any personal stories about anyone in the class or school;

+ feeling free to ask any questions about the topic.

You should make it clear that any pupil who does not follow these ground rules or does not show the kind of behaviour the teacher expects will be removed from the class. You should also make it clear that any pupil who becomes distressed due to the class can remove themselves if they would like to. It is particularly important to mention this before sensitive topics such as abortion and sexual harassment/assault as pupils may have had personal experiences of these issues.

A lot of embarrassment pupils may feel in RSE lessons can stem from the use of proper biologically correct names for sexual activities and body parts. It is not uncommon for pupils (of any age) to laugh or make heckling noises when they hear words such as 'penis', 'vagina', 'oral sex', etc. It is therefore a good practice to inform the class at the beginning of each RSE lesson that you will be using the correct biological names for body parts and sexual acts. Reinforce that the reasons you are doing this is: firstly, to educate everyone on the correct names for body parts and sexual acts as some pupils will only be familiar with slang words and not the correct biological words; secondly, to promote an open atmosphere. These are correct words for body parts and sexual acts: they are nothing to be ashamed of or embarrassed about. Finally, if pupils ever have any worries or problems (in a medical or safeguarding capacity), they can alert an adult they trust with the correct terminology.

Starter or icebreaker activities can be a great technique to promote an open classroom environment and to help pupils overcome any embarrassment they may feel towards RSE.

ACTIVITY 1

I'LL GIVE YOU A MINUTE

This activity provides pupils with an outlet for any embarrassment or laughter they may be suppressing after being told that they will be learning about RSE. You set a timer for 60 seconds, preferably in a place visible to all pupils such as a smartboard. You tell pupils that you are going to give them one minute to say whatever they like to the person next to them/around them about how they feel about the RSE lesson. They can laugh, make any noisy sounds or simply tell the person next to them/around them what they think about the RSE topics. After the minute tell the class that you now expect them to be sensible for the remainder of the lesson. This activity works particularly well with Years 7 and 8.

ACTIVITY 2

SHOUT IT OUT

Similar to *I'll give you a minute*, this activity allows pupils to say silly or slang words at the beginning of the lesson, so that they can then continue the lesson sensibly. Get pupils to shout out any silly or slang words they know to do with body parts, relationships and sex. You can go around the class and ask each pupil to shout out one word or you can ask pupils to volunteer by putting their hand up and then shouting out a word. Do not force pupils to participate if they do not want to. This activity defuses any embarrassment pupils may be feeling towards the RSE lesson.

ACTIVITY 3

RSE WORD ASSOCIATION

This activity is good for specific RSE topics. Pupils can work in pairs or in small groups. Each pair or group gets a piece of A4 paper. They write the topic of the RSE lesson in the middle of the paper such as 'abortion', 'STIs', 'pornography', 'puberty' and then write around the topic all the words and phrases they associate with that topic. Not only does this give pupils time to become comfortable with talking about the topic, but it also provides an opportunity for you to see what knowledge pupils already have on the RSE topic.

✚ CHAPTER 1
SEX

QUESTIONS ASKED IN THIS CHAPTER

1. *Why do people have sex?*
2. *Is first-time sex painful?*
3. *Is masturbating normal?*
4. *How long does sex usually last?*
5. *What is oral sex?*
6. *What is anal sex?*
7. *What is vaginal sex?*
8. *What is sexual touching?*
9. *When should you have sex?*
10. *Can you get pregnant from anal sex?*

TEACHER GUIDANCE

The topic 'sex' when discussed in secondary school will always be met with a few embarrassing laughs or pupils calling out in alarm, especially in Years 7 and 8. It is worth considering that this may be one of the very few times they have ever heard the word 'sex' spoken by an adult. During RSE topics where sex/sexual activities are discussed, pupils ask you 'tester' questions. These are questions pupils will ask to shock you or get a reaction out of you. The reason pupils ask this type of question is because they either find it funny or want to see your reaction before they ask a question that they genuinely want to know about. Needless to say, you should not react to these questions with shock or surprise and answer them as factually as possible.

EXAMPLE TESTER QUESTION

Pupil: *How do you have sex?*

If this question has been asked during a session with Years 7 or 8 and is not relevant to the RSE topic of the lesson, an appropriate response would be:

Teacher: *That's a great question but it's not really relevant to the topic we are currently talking about. If you want to find out about this, you can wait until the end of the lesson and I can talk to you about this. Or I can give you some useful websites where you can find out this information for yourself.*

If this question is asked during a session with Years 10 or 11 and is relevant to the RSE topic of the lesson, then an appropriate response would be:

Teacher: *That's a great question. Which type of sex are you talking about? Vaginal sex, oral sex, anal sex or sexual touching?*

This response shows that the question is valid and clarifies what kind of sexual activity they are talking about. Therefore, you as the teacher can give the correct information.

QUESTIONS

1. WHY DO PEOPLE HAVE SEX?

There are many different reasons why people might have sex. It may be to conceive a baby, or because it feels good and gives them sexual pleasure or as a way to be intimate and close to one another and express their love physically. Even if you have sex with someone you don't love, it is important to remember that you should always have sex with someone you trust and feel comfortable with.

2. IS FIRST-TIME SEX PAINFUL?

First-time sex shouldn't be painful for men or women. You may have heard that you should expect first-time penetrative sex to be painful but actually this is a myth. If you are finding sex painful you need to communicate this to your partner. Painful sex could be a sign that you are not relaxed enough, you are going too fast or it could be related to a health issue. No one should have to experience painful sex.

3. IS MASTURBATING NORMAL?

Masturbating in a private space such as your own bedroom or a locked bathroom at home is completely normal and legal. During puberty boys and girls may get feelings and urges to masturbate. This is completely normal and healthy.

4. HOW LONG DOES SEX USUALLY LAST?

Sex lasts as long as the people who are having sex want it to last! There is no 'normal duration', it's just whatever works for you. However, if you are a man having penetrative sex (oral, anal or vaginal sex) for more than 20–30 minutes you'll need to change condoms as it is likely to tear or break after that duration.

5. WHAT IS ORAL SEX?

Oral sex is when someone uses their mouth or tongue to stimulate a person's penis, vagina or vulva.

6. WHAT IS ANAL SEX?

Anal sex is any sort of touching, kissing or penetration of the anus. People can have anal sex with a penis or by using a sex toy.

7. WHAT IS VAGINAL SEX?

Vaginal sex is any sort of touching or penetration of the vagina. People can have vaginal sex with a penis or by using a sex toy.

8. WHAT IS SEXUAL TOUCHING?

Sexual touching includes any sort of kissing, stoking or rubbing of genitals or erogenous zones for the purpose of arousing someone.

9. WHEN SHOULD YOU HAVE SEX?

The age of consent in the UK for all genders and sexualities is 16. This means if you take part in any sexual activity before the age of 16 it is deemed as illegal (even if you are consenting to it). Even though the age of consent is 16, you do not have to take part in any sexual activity at 16 if you don't want to. You should only take part in sexual activities when you feel ready, comfortable and want to. Friends or a sexual partner should never pressure you into sexual activity.

10. CAN YOU GET PREGNANT FROM ANAL SEX?

There isn't a direct internal path from the anus to the reproductive organs. However there is a small chance you can get pregnant from anal sex if a man and a woman are having unprotected anal sex. This is because the anus is very close to the vagina. So, during ejaculation, if fluid leaks or spills close to the vagina there is a possibility that sperm can reach the egg. If you want to avoid becoming pregnant you should use any contraceptive methods.

SOURCES OF FURTHER INFORMATION

The NHS website – www.nhs.uk

Brook – www.brook.org.uk

FPA – www.fpa.org.uk

Sexwise – www.sexwise.org.uk

The Mix: Sex and Relationships – www.themix.org.uk/sex-and-relationships

✛ CHAPTER 2

CONTRACEPTION

QUESTIONS ASKED IN THIS CHAPTER

1. *How many types of contraception are there?*
2. *What is the combined pill?*
3. *What is the progestogen-only pill?*
4. *What is the contraceptive patch?*
5. *What is the contraceptive injection?*
6. *What is the implant?*
7. *What is the IUS?*
8. *What is the vaginal ring?*
9. *What is a female/internal condom?*
10. *What is an IUD?*
11. *What is a diaphragm or cap?*
12. *Does all contraception stop STIs and pregnancy?*
13. *Where can you get contraception from? Do you have to pay for it?*
14. *How old do you need to be to get contraception?*
15. *Can you take only the morning after pill the morning after you've had sex?*
16. *Is the emergency contraceptive pill the same as an abortion?*
17. *Where can you get the emergency contraceptive pill from?*

⟶

18. *What is a condom?*

19. *How do you check a condom before using it?*

20. *How do you put on a condom?*

21. *Can you be allergic to condoms?*

22. *Which type of contraception is best?*

23. *Does contraception have any side effects?*

TEACHER GUIDANCE

One of the most important points to remember when educating young people on contraception is to refrain from projecting personal biases. For the most part, our knowledge on contraception is based on our own personal experience of sex and relationships. It may be tempting when talking about the contraceptive pill to add: 'My friend's son was conceived while she was on the contraceptive pill' or 'Condoms never really work in my experience'. However well meaning, such comments cross student–teacher boundaries by revealing personal information that is not required. Additionally, it may discourage students from using a particular type of contraception in the future if an unconscious negative bias is introduced.

When discussing contraception, it is important to remember inclusivity. Although the majority of people believe contraception equates to preventing pregnancy, it is important to educate that contraception can also lead to a reduction in STIs. Therefore, it is essential that contraception is discussed for all sexual relationships, that is, heterosexual and LGBTQ+ relationships. Many sexual acts carry a risk of STI transmission. Vaginal sex, anal sex, oral sex, genital to genital touching and sharing sex toys can all lead to STIs if contraception is not used correctly or if it is not used at all.

QUESTIONS

1. HOW MANY TYPES OF CONTRACEPTION ARE THERE?

There are 15 types of contraception available in the UK. These can be categorised into two main groups.

TABLE 2.1 Hormonal contraception

Contraception type	Effectiveness
Combined pill	Between 91 and 99 per cent
Contraceptive injection	Between 94 and 99 per cent
Contraceptive patch	Between 91 and 99 per cent
Emergency contraception pill	Between 97 and 99 per cent
Implant	More than 99 per cent
IUS	More than 99 per cent
Progestogen-only pill	Between 91 and 99 per cent
Vaginal ring	Between 91 and 99 per cent

(NHS Contraception Guide, 2020)

TABLE 2.2 Non-hormonal contraception

Contraception type	Effectiveness
Diaphragm or cap	Between 71 and 96 per cent
Female/internal condoms	Between 79 and 95 per cent
IUD	More than 99 per cent
Male condoms	Between 82 and 98 per cent
Natural family planning/fertility awareness	Between 76 and 99 per cent

(NHS Contraception Guide, 2020)

In addition to these two main groups there are two permanent methods of contraception.

TABLE 2.3 Permanent contraception

Contraception type	Effectiveness
Male sterilisation (vasectomy)	More than 99 per cent
Female sterilisation	More than 99 per cent

(NHS Contraception Guide, 2020)

2. WHAT IS THE COMBINED PILL?

The combined pill contains the hormones progestogen and oestrogen. Releasing both the hormones prevents ovulation. The hormones also cause the lining of the uterus to become thinner so a fertilised egg

19

cannot implant itself. The hormones also thicken the mucus around the cervix making it difficult (but not impossible) for sperm to enter the uterus. The combined pill is taken by the woman daily for 21 days followed by a seven-day break. During this seven-day break a woman may experience a hormonal bleeding. The combined pill has to be taken at the same time each day in order for it to be most effective. If a woman forgets to take the combined pill on any one day of the 21 days, she may not be protected against pregnancy for that pill cycle.

3. WHAT IS THE PROGESTOGEN-ONLY PILL?

The progestogen-only pill (sometimes called the 'mini pill') is similar to the combined pill. The difference however is that as the name implies it only contains the hormone progestogen. When taken, the pill stops ovulation and makes the mucus of the cervix thicker making it difficult (but not impossible) for sperm to enter the uterus. The progestogen-only pill needs to be taken at the same time every day continuously in order for it to be effective. If a woman forgets to take the combined pill one day she may not be protected against pregnancy.

4. WHAT IS THE CONTRACEPTIVE PATCH?

The contraceptive patch is a small 5 cm^2 plaster that is stuck to a woman's body. It can be stuck anywhere (apart from the breasts) and so is discrete if needed. It is sticky and so stays in place while in the shower, bath or swimming pool. The contraceptive patch works by releasing progestogen hormones through the skin, which prevents ovulation. The hormone causes the lining of the uterus to become thinner so a fertilised egg cannot implant itself. The hormones also thicken the mucus around the cervix making it difficult (but not impossible) for sperm to enter the uterus. The contraceptive patch lasts for seven days and then has to be replaced by a new contraceptive patch.

5. WHAT IS THE CONTRACEPTIVE INJECTION?

The contraceptive injection contains the hormone progestogen and is administered by a doctor or nurse into a woman's arm or bottom. Once injected it works by releasing the hormone progestogen which prevents ovulation. The hormone causes the lining of the uterus to become thinner so a fertilised egg cannot implant itself. The hormone also thickens the mucus around the cervix, making it difficult (but not impossible) for sperm to enter the uterus. The contraceptive injection protects against pregnancy for up to 13 weeks.

6. WHAT IS THE IMPLANT?

The implant is a 4 cm plastic rod that is inserted by a doctor or nurse into a woman's forearm. It generally cannot be seen but a woman can feel it under her skin. The implant works by releasing progestogen hormone that prevents ovulation. The hormone causes the lining of the uterus to become thinner, so a fertilised egg cannot implant itself. The hormones also thicken the mucus around the cervix making it difficult (but not impossible) for sperm to enter the uterus. The implant once inserted protects the woman from pregnancy for up to three years and can be removed at any time by a doctor.

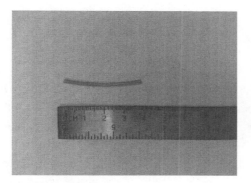

Figure 2.1 Implant

7. WHAT IS THE IUS?

The intra-uterine system (IUS) is a small plastic device that is fitted into the uterus by a doctor or nurse. The IUS works by releasing the progestogen hormone that prevents ovulation. The hormone causes the lining of the uterus to become thinner, so a fertilised egg cannot implant itself. The hormones also thicken the mucus around the cervix, making it difficult (but not impossible) for sperm to enter the uterus. Once inserted, the IUS protects the woman from pregnancy for up to five years and can be removed at any time by a doctor.

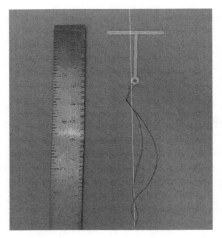

Figure 2.2 IUS

8. WHAT IS THE VAGINAL RING?

The vaginal ring is a small plastic ring that can be inserted into the vagina by a woman herself. The vaginal ring works by releasing the progestogen hormone that prevents ovulation. The hormone causes the lining

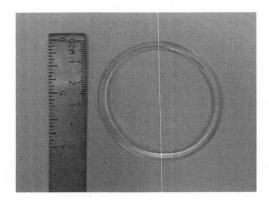

Figure 2.3 Vaginal ring

of the uterus to become thinner, so a fertilised egg cannot implant itself. The hormones also thicken the mucus around the cervix, making it difficult (but not impossible) for sperm to enter the uterus. Once inserted the vaginal ring stays inside the vagina for three weeks. It is then removed for seven days and a new vaginal ring is inserted after this break.

9. WHAT IS A FEMALE/INTERNAL CONDOM?

The female/internal condom works in the same way as a male condom. It acts as a physical barrier to prevent sperm from reaching an egg. It stops sexual fluids being exchanged with the partner and hence prevents STIs. The female/internal condom can be inserted into the vagina or anus. Each female condom must be used only once during sexual activity.

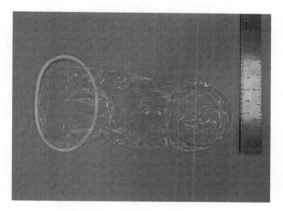

Figure 2.4 Female/internal condom

10. WHAT IS AN IUD?

The intra-uterine device (IUD) is a small plastic device attached to a thin strip of copper that is fitted into the uterus by a doctor or nurse. It prevents pregnancy because copper is toxic to sperm and kills them. Once inserted the IUD can protect the woman from pregnancy for up to ten years and can be removed at any time by a doctor or nurse.

11. WHAT IS A DIAPHRAGM OR CAP?

The diaphragm or cap is a small dome-shaped device that acts as a physical barrier during sex. It prevents pregnancy by covering the entrance to the cervix and stops sperm from meeting the egg. Before being used for the first time, a woman needs to be examined by a doctor or nurse to ensure that the correct size diaphragm is used. Once the correct size has been ascertained then the woman can insert the diaphragm herself. The diaphragm or cap needs to be used with spermicide gel. After sex, the diaphragm or cap needs to be left inside the vagina for six hours and then removed and washed. After this it can be reused.

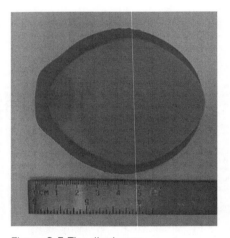

Figure 2.5 The diaphragm

12. DOES ALL CONTRACEPTION STOP STIs AND PREGNANCY?

Contraception, if used correctly, is almost 100 per cent effective at preventing unwanted pregnancy. However, only condoms (male and female) can protect you from STIs. That is why it is crucial that if a male and female are engaging in sexual activity, even if the woman is on hormonal contraception like the implant or combined pill, you also use a condom to prevent STIs.

24

13. WHERE CAN YOU GET CONTRACEPTION FROM? DO YOU HAVE TO PAY FOR IT?

You can obtain most forms of contraception from your local doctor or local sexual health clinic. All forms of contraception are free on the National Health Service (NHS). Many types of council have their own free condom distribution scheme for under 18s and in some colleges and universities condoms are available for free from student services. You can get condoms from many other places such as pharmacies, supermarkets and online; however, you do have to pay for condoms in these circumstances.

NOTE TO TEACHERS

It is worth researching what condom distribution schemes are available in your local area.

---

14. HOW OLD DO YOU NEED TO BE TO GET CONTRACEPTION?

The age of consent in the UK is 16; however, you can legally access contraception from the age of 13 if you can demonstrate that you understand what it is used for and how it works. You will normally need to go to a doctor or sexual health clinic to obtain contraception. It is your legal right to access confidential sexual health advice and contraception services from the age of 13 without your parents' knowledge and permission if you need it.

NOTE TO TEACHERS

You might want to point out to students that there are medical reasons to use hormonal contraception. For example, if a young woman experiences painful and heavy periods then she may be put on the combined pill to help regulate her periods and make them less painful.

---

15. CAN YOU ONLY TAKE THE MORNING AFTER PILL THE MORNING AFTER YOU'VE HAD SEX?

This is actually a common myth. Emergency contraception or 'the morning after pill' can be taken up to five days after unprotected sex.

There are two types of emergency contraception pills:

+ Levonelle: this can be taken up to 72 hours after unprotected sex.

+ EllaOne: this can be taken up to 120 hours after unprotected sex.

In order to be effective, it is important that emergency contraception is taken as soon as possible after unprotected sex. The IUD (copper coil) can also be used as a form of emergency contraception up to five days after unprotected sex; but in this case the IUD must be inserted by a doctor.

16. IS THE EMERGENCY CONTRACEPTIVE PILL THE SAME AS AN ABORTION?

This is a common misconception. The emergency contraceptive pill is not an abortion. The emergency contraceptive pill works by delaying the release of an egg from the ovaries (ovulation). This is because sperm can survive in the vagina and uterus for up to five days after unprotected sex. If there is no egg for the sperm to fertilise because the emergency contraceptive pill has delayed ovulation, then a pregnancy cannot begin. If fertilisation has already happened, the emergency contraceptive pill will not work. It cannot affect or harm a fertilised egg.

17. WHERE CAN YOU GET THE EMERGENCY CONTRACEPTIVE PILL FROM?

You can get the emergency contraceptive pill for free, even if you are under the age of 16, from sexual health clinics, some GPs, some A&E departments, most NHS walk-in centres and pharmacies.

If you are over the age of 16, you can buy the contraceptive pill from most pharmacies. Depending on which emergency contraceptive pill you buy, the cost will be between £16 and £32.

18. WHAT IS A CONDOM?

A condom is a thin barrier made of latex (or non-latex rubber) that can be worn over the penis during sexual activity. When used correctly, it can prevent STI transmission and unwanted pregnancies.

19. HOW DO YOU CHECK A CONDOM BEFORE USING IT?

Before using a condom, check the expiry date on the back of the condom wrapper. Firstly, if the expiry date has passed, then do not use it as it is more likely to break or tear. Secondly, check if the condom has the CE mark on the wrapper as this means the condom has been made to the correct standards and has been quality checked. Poorly made condoms will not have this mark on the wrapper. Finally, check if the condom is neither damaged nor has any holes. An easy way to do this is to push the condom to one side of the wrapper. If the condom is not damaged, you should be able to feel an air bubble. If the condom is damaged or has a hole in it, you will not be able to feel an air bubble.

20. HOW DO YOU PUT ON A CONDOM?

NOTE TO TEACHERS

The best way to teach students correct condom use is by using a condom demonstrator. For teachers who do not feel comfortable doing this, you can find online educational videos or tell students the following step-by-step guidelines.

Step 1: After you have checked the outside wrapper of a condom carefully open it making sure not to tear it with your fingernails. Make sure the condom is not inside out. If the condom is inside out it may not unroll over the penis correctly.

NOTE TO TEACHERS

Depending on the age group, a good visual tool to get students to remember which way around a condom should be is by telling them the condom should look like a sombrero hat if it is in correct position and if it is inside out it should look like the top of a baby's bottle.

Step 2: Pinch the top of the condom between your finger and thumb. This will prevent any air bubbles at the top of the condom (an air bubble could cause the condom to break during sex).

Step 3: Place the condom at the head of the erect penis. Then roll the condom down the length of the penis while still pinching the top of the condom. Make sure the condom is secure.

Step 4: After you finish having sex hold the condom in place and remove the condom while the penis is still erect. Check the condom has not leaked and then tie a knot at the end of the condom to prevent any fluid leaking out.

Step 5: Wrap the condom in a tissue and thrown it in the bin. Never reuse a condom and never throw a condom away down a toilet.

21. CAN YOU BE ALLERGIC TO CONDOMS?

Some people do have a latex allergy, and many condom brands now offer latex-free condoms. Free condom distribution schemes also usually supply latex-free condoms.

22. WHICH TYPE OF CONTRACEPTION IS BEST?

There is no perfect type of contraception for everyone. Women who use hormonal contraception can have varied experiences with the same type of contraception. It is important to try out different contraception methods to find out what works best for you.

23. DOES CONTRACEPTION HAVE ANY SIDE EFFECTS?

Some (but not all) women who use hormonal contraception can experience mild to severe side effects such as bleeding, acne, nausea, weight gain/loss, loss of sex drive and headaches. If you obtain contraception from a sexual health clinic or local doctor you will be advised about possible side effects. If the side effects become distressing or severely interfere with your day-to-day life, please speak to your doctor or consider changing the type of contraception you use.

SOURCES OF FURTHER INFORMATION

Brook – www.brook.org.uk

Contraception Choices – www.contraceptionchoices.org

FPA – www.fpa.org.uk

The NHS Website – www.nhs.uk

The Mix – www.themix.org.uk

✚ CHAPTER 3
RELATIONSHIPS

QUESTIONS ASKED IN THIS CHAPTER

1. *Should I spend all my time with my partner?*

2. *Is it bad if you do not like your partner's friends?*

3. *If my partner and I keep arguing, should we break up?*

4. *If my partner buys me expensive gifts, should I do anything they ask me?*

5. *What is relationship abuse?*

6. *What are the types of relationship abuse?*

7. *What age should I start committing to a relationship?*

8. *How can I communicate well with my partner?*

9. *If I am in a long-distance relationship, how can we be intimate?*

10. *Is it normal to meet romantic/sexual partners online?*

11. *Can I be in a relationship with two people at once?*

TEACHER GUIDANCE

It can be easy to be dismissive of the importance of relationships for pupils. Family relationships and friendships are extremely important in shaping a pupil's life while also providing a support network for that pupil. Early romantic and sexual relationships are also significant for pupils as they shape future relationship behaviours. It is important to remember that a lot of peer-on-peer relationship abuse can happen within these early romantic and sexual relationships as pupils are still negotiating boundaries and forging their understanding of consent. This is why early relationship education is vital for secondary school pupils as it provides them with the understanding of what a healthy and unhealthy relationship looks like.

QUESTIONS

1. SHOULD I SPEND ALL MY TIME WITH MY PARTNER?

At the beginning of a new relationship, you may want to spend all your time with your new partner because the relationship is new and exciting. This is a normal and healthy reaction. However, it is important that you remember to see your friends, family and have some time alone to yourself as well. Your friends and family may feel upset and forgotten if you do not see them very often once you get into a relationship. So, it is important to consider their feelings as well. It is also worth considering that your partner may not want to spend all their time with you. This does not mean they do not want to be in a relationship with you but that they need time in their own space with their friends or family. Part of being in a healthy relationship is finding the right balance between spending time together and spending time apart.

2. IS IT BAD IF YOU DO NOT LIKE YOUR PARTNER'S FRIENDS?

In a world of 7.8 billion people, there are going to be some people you just do not get on with. Some people are fine with their partner not liking their friends but for some people it will upset them. If your partner is upset with you not liking their friends, then make sure you take time to communicate and tell your partner why you do not like them. Then your partner may understand your perspective more. Even if you do not like your partner's friends, do not force your partner to stop being friends with them. Your partner can choose whoever they want to be friends with, and you must respect this. If you do not, this can be a sign of emotionally abusive and manipulative behaviour.

3. IF MY PARTNER AND I KEEP ARGUING, SHOULD WE BREAK UP?

It is normal to have disagreements in any relationship. Everyone is different and there are some things that people are bound to disagree on. A healthy relationship is one where partners can discuss their problems calmly and reasonably. This means listening to the other person's point of view and compromising with your partner. There may be things that you cannot compromise on and then you have to decide whether or not this will be a problem in your relationship you can accept or whether you feel it would be better to end the relationship. If an argument ever becomes physically violent or emotionally abusive, this is a warning sign of relationship abuse. No one should ever have to put up with this in a relationship.

4. IF MY PARTNER BUYS ME EXPENSIVE GIFTS, SHOULD I DO ANYTHING THEY ASK ME?

Sometimes in relationships partners will buy each other gifts, whether this is for an occasion such as a birthday, anniversary or seasonal holiday or when you do not expect it, for no reason. This can be a great gesture and make you feel happy within the relationship. However, just because your partner buys you gifts it does not give them the right to control you and ask you to do things for them. If your partner starts expecting you to do things you do not want to do because they have bought you gifts, this can be a sign of controlling and coercive behaviour. This could then turn into relationship abuse. If you are ever worried about this, it is important to talk to someone you trust who can support you.

5. WHAT IS RELATIONSHIP ABUSE?

Relationship abuse can occur within any type of relationship. This includes a relationship between a parent and child, friends or in a romantic or sexual relationship. There are different types of relationship abuse including sexual, physical, emotional, psychological and financial. The shared experience of victims in an abusive relationship is that they feel unsafe, frightened and not free to be themselves.

6. WHAT ARE THE TYPES OF RELATIONSHIP ABUSE?

Relationship abuse can occur in any relationship. This includes a relationship between friends, family and parent–child relationship, professional relationship as well as a romantic or sexual relationship. There are many different types of relationship abuse, but the main types are as follows.

+ **Physical abuse**: hitting, punching, biting or pushing someone.

+ **Emotional abuse**: calling someone names, insulting them, swearing at them and making someone feel worthless.

+ **Psychological abuse**: ignoring someone's feelings, making threats, gaslighting and never allowing someone to be right.

+ **Sexual abuse:** forcing someone to engage in sexual activity, showing someone explicit sexual images or videos without consent, forcing someone to stop using contraception, violent sexual activity.

+ **Financial abuse**: controls how you spend money, steals money from you, refuses to let you work, makes you beg for money.

Relationship abuse can happen to anyone regardless of age or gender and is never acceptable.

7. WHAT AGE SHOULD I START COMMITTING TO A RELATIONSHIP?

There is no right age to start committing to a relationship. It is important that you feel comfortable and ready before you enter a romantic relationship. You should never feel forced or pressured to enter into

34

a romantic relationship that you do not want to. Many people have successful romantic relationships from secondary school onwards. It is worth remembering that if you want to begin a sexual relationship under the age of 16, there are laws to consider.

8. HOW CAN I COMMUNICATE WELL WITH MY PARTNER?

Communication, while sometimes difficult, is a key element of any successful and healthy relationship. The best way to practice good communication with your partner is to always be completely open and honest about how you are feeling and things that are bothering you. Do not suppress any worries or problems you have in the hope that they will just disappear. Your partner will not know your worries or problems unless you communicate them. Also, by suppressing worries and problems you are more likely to have a bad argument with your partner when you finally express yourself.

9. IF I AM IN A LONG-DISTANCE RELATIONSHIP, HOW CAN WE BE INTIMATE?

Being in a long-distance relationship can be difficult, and especially when you cannot be physical with them. However, intimacy does not have to depend on whether your partner is geographically close to you. There are many ways you can be close and intimate with your partner without being physically close. A great way to maintain intimacy is to schedule a specific time to talk via phone or video chat. This could be a specific time every day or every few days or once a week. By having scheduled calls or video chats, this shows that your partner and you are making time to communicate and develop your relationship.

10. IS IT NORMAL TO MEET ROMANTIC/ SEXUAL PARTNERS ONLINE?

Today, many relationships start by meeting people online, via dating websites or dating apps. It is always important to remember safety rules when dating online. Some dating websites and apps have age restrictions on them due to potentially graphic content. It is also very important to consider your personal safety when meeting with someone you have met online for the first time. Meet in a public area and always tell a trusted friend where and what time you are meeting.

11. CAN I BE IN A RELATIONSHIP WITH TWO PEOPLE AT ONCE?

Some people enjoy dating or having a romantic or sexual relationship with more than one person at a time. These are called non-monogamous relationships. These relationships are very common in different cultures and countries around the world. If you want to be in a non-monogamous relationship, the most important thing to consider is communication and honesty with your partners. It is important that you tell people you date/begin a relationship with that you are in a non-monogamous relationship. Consent and contraception should also be discussed within non-monogamous relationships.

SOURCES OF FURTHER INFORMATION

Brook – www.brook.org.uk

Childline – www.childline.org.uk

Love is Respect – www.loveisrespect.org

SH:24 – www.sh24.org.uk

The Mix – www.themix.org.uk

✛ CHAPTER 4
SEXUALLY TRANSMITTED INFECTIONS

QUESTIONS ASKED IN THIS CHAPTER

1. *What does STI stand for?*

2. *What types of STIs are there?*

3. *Can all STIs be cured?*

4. *If it hurts when you pee, is it an STI?*

5. *How do you get an STI?*

6. *Can you catch an STI from a toilet seat?*

7. *Is AIDS an STI?*

8. *Can you get an STI through kissing someone on the lips?*

9. *If you do not have pubic hair, does that mean you cannot catch pubic lice?*

10. *How old do you have to be to get an STI test?*

11. *Where can you get an STI test?*

12. *How long should you wait after unprotected sex to get an STI test?*

13. *Can someone tell I have an STI by looking at me?*

14. *Can you get an STI from oral sex?*

15. *Can you get an STI from masturbating?*

$\longrightarrow$

16. *What happens during an STI test at a sexual health clinic/GP?*

17. *How does a home STI testing kit work?*

18. *If I have an STI, do I have to tell people?*

19. *Can I get into trouble if I give someone an STI?*

20. *Is thrush an STI?*

TEACHER GUIDANCE

STIs are still stigmatised within our society. People also associate STIs with shame and therefore do not get tested for them as often as they should or do not understand how or where to get tested. The taboo around STIs stems from two factors. Firstly, STIS are not taught properly in schools, allowing myths and misconceptions to circulate. Secondly, when they are covered in the curriculum, they are taught in a way that promotes scaremongering and actually fails to include practical information about how to/where to get an STI test, what happens during an STI test and also information about testing windows. STIs are nothing to be scared or ashamed of but anyone who is sexually active need to be aware of them.

QUESTIONS

1. WHAT DOES STI STAND FOR?

STI stands for 'sexually transmitted infection'. You may hear STIs are sometimes referred to as STDs (sexually transmitted diseases) but this is now an incorrect and out-of-date term. STDs was changed to STIs to reflect the fact that all STIs are treatable.

2. WHAT TYPES OF STIs ARE THERE?

There are three groups of STIs: bacterial, viral and parasitic.

+ Bacterial STIs include gonorrhea, syphilis, chlamydia and trichomoniasis.

38

+ Viral STIs include HIV, genital warts and herpes.

+ Parasitic STIs include pubic lice (sometimes known as crabs).

3. CAN ALL STIs BE CURED?

Not every STI can be cured but all STIs are treatable. Bacterial STIs like chlamydia and gonorrhea can be cured with antibiotics. Viral STIs like HIV and herpes cannot be cured, which means the virus always remains in your body. However, there is a treatment in the form of anti-retroviral drugs that you can take to suppress the symptoms of these STIs. Parasitic STIs such as pubic lice can easily be treated and cured with an insecticide shampoo.

4. IF IT HURTS WHEN YOU PEE, IS IT AN STI?

Pain when urinating can be a symptom of many things like a urinary tract infection or cystitis as well as an STI. If you are ever worried about a symptom the best thing to do is see your GP or get an STI test.

5. HOW DO YOU GET AN STI?

STIs can be transmitted mainly through exchange of bodily fluids such as semen, vaginal fluids and blood. Some STIs like genital warts and herpes can be transmitted through close genital to genital contact, which means you do not need to have penetrative sex to be at the risk of contracting these STIs. Finally, pubic lice can be transmitted through close body contact as the lice can crawl from one person to another person. In very rare cases, you can be at risk from pubic lice if you share towels or bedding with someone who is infected with them.

6. CAN YOU CATCH AN STI FROM A TOILET SEAT?

Absolutely not; this is a common myth. Most STIs are transmitted through bodily fluids or skin to skin genital contact. Bodily fluids like semen and vaginal fluids left on a toilet seat cannot get into the body by a person just sitting on a toilet seat.

7. IS AIDS AN STI?

This is a common misconception. AIDs is what HIV can progress to if HIV is not treated correctly. People who are HIV positive that are on the correct medication and undergo regular health checks will not develop AIDs.

8. CAN YOU GET AN STI THROUGH KISSING SOMEONE ON THE LIPS?

Although some STIs are transmitted through bodily fluids, this does not include saliva. The only STI you can get through kissing is oral herpes. Herpes is transmitted through skin to skin contact, so if you are kissing and therefore having skin to skin contact with someone who has a herpes sore on their face then it is possible to contract herpes.

9. IF YOU DO NOT HAVE PUBIC HAIR, DOES THAT MEAN YOU CANNOT CATCH PUBIC LICE?

If you remove your pubic hair you might think that you have less chances of catching public lice. However, pubic lice only need a small part of the hair follicle to lay their eggs and live on a person's body. Pubic lice can also crawl to hair on other parts of your body to live such as underarm hair and eyelashes.

10. HOW OLD DO YOU HAVE TO BE TO GET AN STI TEST?

There is no age requirement for you to get an STI test. You can access STI testing services at any age even if you are under the age of 16.

11. WHERE CAN YOU GET AN STI TEST?

You can get an STI test from your GP or from a specialist sexual health clinic. In some parts of the UK, you can even get free home STI testing kits posted to you. This means you can take an STI test in the comfort of your own home without going to your GP or a sexual health clinic.

12. HOW LONG SHOULD YOU WAIT AFTER UNPROTECTED SEX TO GET AN STI TEST?

The time you should wait after you have an STI test depends on the type of STIs you are testing for:

+ For bacterial STIs like chlamydia and gonorrhoea you need to wait two weeks for an accurate result.

+ For viral STIs like HIV, syphilis and hepatitis some rapid tests give an accurate result after four weeks. Non-rapid tests must be taken 12 weeks after unprotected sex.

13. CAN SOMEONE TELL I HAVE AN STI BY LOOKING AT ME?

You cannot always tell someone has an STI just by looking at them. Many people do not present any symptoms when they have an STI and are not aware of themselves that they have one.

14. CAN YOU GET AN STI FROM ORAL SEX?

Yes, you can catch an STI during oral sex. This is why it is important to use contraception when taking part in oral sex. If you are performing oral sex on a man, then you can use a condom that will act as a barrier to protect you from STIs. You can purchase different flavoured condoms specifically for this purpose and to make oral sex more enjoyable. If you are performing oral sex on a female's genitals or on someone's anus you should use an oral dam. This is a small, thin square of latex which you can hold in place over a female's genitals or someone's anus which can act as a barrier to protect you from STIs.

41

15. CAN YOU GET AN STI FROM MASTURBATING?

You cannot get an STI from masturbating on your own. You might have heard that masturbating on your own will give you an STI, but this is a myth. There is a risk of getting an STI if you are masturbating or sexually touching a partner and fluids like vaginal fluids or semen are transferred.

16. WHAT HAPPENS DURING AN STI TEST AT A SEXUAL HEALTH CLINIC/GP?

When you go for an STI test, the first thing that will happen is the doctor or nurse will ask you a few personal questions. This will include how old you are, the date of your last STI test (if you have had an STI test before), when you last had sex, the type of sex you had and who you have sex with (males or females). You may find these questions uncomfortable or personal but they are just trying to work out what kind of test to give you. Remember the medical professional is not going to judge you and whatever you tell them will be kept confidential.

You will then have to either provide a urine sample or vaginal swab if you are being tested for bacterial STIs like chlamydia. Most of the time you will be able to provide these samples in private by yourself. If you have had unprotected oral or anal sex and would like to test these areas for bacterial STIs, you'll have to provide a swab for these areas as well. The medical professional will then take a blood sample from your arm. This is to test for HIV, syphilis and hepatitis.

If you have experienced symptoms of an STI such as lumps on your genitals or unusual discharge, the medical professional may ask to examine your penis or vulva.

17. HOW DOES A HOME STI TESTING KIT WORK?

Many health services offer free home STI testing kits. You need to order one on the health provider website and answer a health questionnaire. The questionnaire will ask you personal questions like when did you last have sex and with whom did you have sex with. They can decide what kind of test to send you with the answers they receive for these questions. The test will be sent to the address you supply online. It does not have to be your home address if you are worried about your parents finding out. Inside the test you have to provide a swab or a urine sample depending on what area you are testing. You may also have to provide a small blood sample. There will be instructions within the testing kit to help you. Once you have provided your samples you post the testing kit back to the health provider and you will get your results text to you within a few weeks. Some health services offer results as quickly as five days. If you receive a positive test result, someone from the health service will contact you to discuss treatment options with you.

18. IF I HAVE AN STI, DO I HAVE TO TELL PEOPLE?

Your STI status is confidential between you and your relevant medical professional. However, contacting past partners to inform them that you have an STI is considered an ethical, mature and responsible thing to do. If you feel uncomfortable doing this you can inform the sexual health clinic where you are receiving treatment and they'll be able to anonymously inform previous sexual partners for you.

19. CAN I GET INTO TROUBLE IF I GIVE SOMEONE AN STI?

If you knowingly infect someone with STI (as in, you knew you had an STI and you still had unprotected sex) you can be taken to court. You can be faced with very serious criminal charges if you knowingly transmit HIV to someone.

20. IS THRUSH AN STI?

Thrush is a common yeast infection. It is not an STI but sex can trigger it and it can be passed on sometimes through vaginal sex. Thrush can cause uncomfortable symptoms in men and women such as itching and irritation around the vagina or penis, discharge from the penis or vagina that looks like cottage cheese and soreness when trying to urinate. Thrush can be treated very easily with anti-fungal medication from your GP.

SOURCES OF FURTHER INFORMATION

Brook – www.brook.org.uk

The NHS Website – www.nhs.uk

Sexwise – www.sexwise.org.uk

SH:24 – www.sh24.org.uk

Terrence Higgins Trust – www.tht.org.uk

✚ CHAPTER 5
PUBERTY

QUESTIONS ASKED IN THIS CHAPTER

1. *Are spontaneous erections normal?*

2. *What are wet dreams?*

3. *What age do boys/girls start puberty?*

4. *Is it normal to feel sad/angry/irritable for no reason during puberty?*

5. *When do boys/girls stop puberty?*

6. *What physical changes happen during puberty?*

7. *What mental changes happen during puberty?*

8. *What age should I start growing breasts?*

9. *Is it normal to have pubic hair?*

10. *Should I start removing my body hair when I reach puberty?*

11. *Is it okay if my breasts do not look the same as everyone else's breasts?*

12. *Why is it important to keep clean during puberty?*

13. *Why do I sweat more?*

14. *Is it normal to get spots over your body as well as your face?*

TEACHER GUIDANCE

When teaching about puberty it is important to try not to focus on our own personal experiences. While empathy and understanding is important, such comments about how we experienced puberty cross pupil–teacher boundaries. It can also be damaging for pupils to compare their experiences of puberty to yours as it may make them worry. For example, if a teacher states in front of the class that they started having periods when they were 14 but there are some 15 year-olds in the class who haven't started their periods it may make these pupils worry.

QUESTIONS

1. ARE SPONTANEOUS ERECTIONS NORMAL?

During puberty it is completely normal for boys to experience spontaneous erections. This is when blood rushes to the penis and makes the penis go hard and stiff. Sometimes boys will get erections when they think about sex or a person they find attractive. Other times boys will experience erections when they are not expecting it. Although you may find this embarrassing, it is completely natural and nothing to worry about.

2. WHAT ARE WET DREAMS?

A wet dream is when boys ejaculate sperm out of their penis involuntarily when they are sleeping. It may be due to dreaming about sexual images when they are sleeping. Some boys find waking up to find they have had a wet dream embarrassing, but it is completely normal for some boys to experience them during puberty.

3. WHAT AGE DO BOYS/GIRLS START PUBERTY?

The average age girls start puberty is around 11 years old, while the average age boys start puberty is around 13 years old. Puberty can begin a few years before or after this.

4. IS IT NORMAL TO FEEL SAD/ANGRY/ IRRITABLE FOR NO REASON DURING PUBERTY?

During puberty, hormones can cause you to experience strong emotions like sadness, anger and annoyance out of the blue. Even if you do not know what has triggered these emotions, they can still feel very intense and overwhelming. You may find yourself arguing with friends and family members more often as a result of these emotions. Try to explain to them how you are feeling so they can understand and support you. If you are constantly experiencing low moods, talk to an adult you trust so they can support you.

5. WHEN DO BOYS/GIRLS STOP PUBERTY?

On average, puberty ends for boys and girls between the ages of 17 and 19 in the UK. Some changes that happen during puberty can occur later.

6. WHAT PHYSICAL CHANGES HAPPEN DURING PUBERTY?

Boys and girls experience many different physical changes during puberty.

Boys:

+ penis and testicles grow larger;
+ chest and shoulders become broader;
+ voice deepens;
+ may start to get erections.

Girls:

+ hips start to widen;
+ labia and clitoris start to grow larger;
+ periods start;
+ breasts start to develop and grow;
+ may experience vaginal discharge.

Both:

+ grow taller;

+ gain weight;

+ hair grows and thickens on arms, legs, under arms and around the genitals;

+ start to sweat more;

+ may get spots on face and body;

+ hair and skin may get oily.

7. WHAT MENTAL CHANGES HAPPEN DURING PUBERTY?

You may find the changes that are happening to your body exciting and interesting. However, sometimes the changes that happen to your body can make you feel anxious and angry. During puberty your body changes from a child into an adult; this includes your mind maturing as well. It is completely normal during puberty for you to feel anxious, sad, angry or pressured. You may also start feeling attracted to people. This can be exciting or confusing. It is important to remember that whatever you are feeling is valid and normal. However, just because intense emotions and mood swings are common during puberty doesn't mean you should struggle with them on your own. If you find your emotions overwhelming it is important to talk to an adult you trust for support.

8. WHAT AGE SHOULD I START GROWING BREASTS?

Girls can start developing breasts any time between the ages of 8 and 13, although some girls do not develop breasts until much later. Breasts can take up to five years to fully grow and develop.

9. IS IT NORMAL TO HAVE PUBIC HAIR?

Pubic hair is the name of the hair that grows around a person's genitals. Boys and girls both grow pubic hair. You may have heard some people describe pubic hair as 'dirty' or 'unclean'. This is a common myth. Pubic hair is healthy as it provides an extra barrier to protect your genitals from bacteria. Some people choose to remove their pubic hair. This is completely your personal choice. No one should ever force you to remove your pubic hair if you do not want to.

10. SHOULD I START REMOVING MY BODY HAIR WHEN I REACH PUBERTY?

During puberty some types of body hair grow more and thicker such as leg hair, underarm hair and pubic hair. Some people (girls and boys) decide they would rather remove this hair. You can remove hair in lots of different ways, such as shaving, hair removal cream or waxing. It is important to remember that removing body hair is a personal choice and no one should ever pressure you into removing your body hair.

11. IS IT OKAY IF MY BREASTS DO NOT LOOK THE SAME AS EVERYONE ELSE'S BREASTS?

Breasts come in all shapes and sizes. Especially during puberty when breasts are developing at a very fast rate, your breasts can change in size and shape every few months. Even after puberty has finished it is common for one breast to be slighty bigger than the other or for one breast to be a different shape to the other. The size and shape of your breasts can also change during your menstrual cycle.

12. WHY IS IT IMPORTANT TO KEEP CLEAN DURING PUBERTY?

It is especially important to wash regularly and keep clean during puberty. This is because the hormones that cause your body to change also can make your body smell. Shower every day, wear clean clothes and use deodorant and/or antiperspirants to stop sweat smelling. It is also very important that you wash your genitals regularly. You do not need expensive or highly perfumed soap to wash your genitals, as warm water and unscented soap is all you need. If you have a foreskin gently pull it to wash under it to stop it from smelling.

13. WHY DO I SWEAT MORE?

During puberty your sweat glands become more active causing you to sweat more. This is why it is very important to keep clean by washing regularly and by using deodorant and/or antiperspirant.

14. IS IT NORMAL TO GET SPOTS OVER YOUR BODY AS WELL AS YOUR FACE?

The hormones that cause puberty changes can also make your skin oily. Oily skin can lead to spots. Most people will get spots on their face, neck and chest but you can get spots anywhere on your body. It is important to not squeeze or pick spots even if they annoy you and you want to get rid of them. Most spots will disappear on their own within a couple of weeks. If the number of spots you have upsets you or if your spots do not go away on their own you can see your GP who can give you special antibiotic cream to get rid of them.

SOURCES OF FURTHER INFORMATION

Beat – www.beateatingdisorders.org.uk

Brook – www.brook.org.uk

Family Lives – www.familylives.org.uk

The Mix – www.themix.org.uk

✚ CHAPTER 6
PERIODS

QUESTIONS ASKED IN THIS CHAPTER

1. *What is a period?*

2. *Can you have vaginal sex on your period?*

3. *What is TSS (toxic shock syndrome)?*

4. *What period products can I use?*

5. *What is PMS?*

6. *Is my period supposed to hurt this much?*

7. *What can I do to help my period pain?*

8. *What age do periods start?*

9. *What age do periods end?*

10. *How long does my period last each cycle?*

11. *My period blood is darker: what does that mean?*

12. *Sometimes I see clumps in my period blood: is that normal?*

13. *How much blood do I lose during my period?*

14. *Can I get pregnant on my period?*

15. *Can I go swimming during my period?*

16. *What is the menopause?*

17. *What are irregular periods?*

$\longrightarrow$

18. *What can make my period late?*

19. *What is period poverty?*

20. *Can you delay your period if you do not want to have it during a holiday?*

TEACHER GUIDANCE

You would not think it, but even today there is still an awful lot of shame and stigma around periods and menstruation. Pupils experiencing their periods may be teased by their peers, and may feel the need to hide period products like sanitary towels and tampons as they go to the toilet. A lot of this is due to a lack of education and misconceptions around periods. The idea of a period to some teenagers (and adults) still evokes disgust. A thorough education about periods and menstruation should eliminate these societal ideas.

Period and menstruation education should not only focus on the biological aspects of the menstrual cycle and reproduction, but also consider and teach about the social aspects of periods such as mental health changes as a side effect of PMS, period bullying and issues surrounding period poverty. Some schools make the mistake of separating pupils and deeming period education not necessary for male pupils to learn about. To promote inclusivity and understanding, it is vital that pupils who do not experience periods, for example, those who have been assigned male at birth, are also included in this comprehensive periods and menstruation education.

QUESTIONS

1. WHAT IS A PERIOD?

A period is a more common term for 'menstrual bleeding'. Between the ages of 8 and 16 girls will start releasing an egg from their ovary. This is called ovulation and happens every 28–35 days. Once an egg is released it travels to the uterus via the fallopian tubes. If the egg has been fertilised by a sperm in the fallopian tubes it will imbed in the lining of the uterus wall. The uterus prepares for the possibility of this happening by building up its uterus wall with a thick layer of spongy tissue. If an egg is not fertilised or does not implant in the uterus lining, then this thick layer of spongy tissue is not needed, and the uterus gets rid of this lining by contracting the muscles of the uterus wall, expelling the thick layer of spongy tissue out of the uterus and out of the vagina. When the lining comes out of the vagina it looks like blood. This is your period or 'menstrual bleeding'.

2. CAN YOU HAVE VAGINAL SEX ON YOUR PERIOD?

Yes, you can have vaginal sex on your period. Choosing to have sex on your period is completely the personal choice of the woman who is on her period. Some women prefer not to have sex on their periods as it can prove to be too uncomfortable or painful. Other women like having sex on their period as it can help to alleviate PMS. Having sex on your period does not eliminate the risk of pregnancy or STI transmission so it is important to use contraception if you are having sex on your period.

3. WHAT IS TSS (TOXIC SHOCK SYNDROME)?

TSS is a serious infection that can sometimes be fatal if not treated quickly. TSS can be caused by not using tampons correctly. To avoid TSS it is vital that you always wash your hands before inserting and removing a tampon. Use a tampon with the lowest absorbency suitable for your period and change your tampon frequently every four to eight hours.

4. WHAT PERIOD PRODUCTS CAN I USE?

There are two types of products available: re-usable and one-time use only products. Tampons and sanitary towels are both one-time use only. However, menstrual cups, fabric sanitary towels and period underwear are all reusable and can last for years if they are cleaned/washed properly.

5. WHAT IS PMS?

PMS stands for premenstrual syndrome and is the name of the mental and physical symptoms a woman can experience shortly before and during her period. Each woman may experience PMS differently, but common symptoms are:

+ mood swings;

+ feeling sad, weepy, angry, or irritable;

+ feeling tired;

+ feeling anxious;

+ bloating;

+ abdominal cramps and stomach aches;

+ increased or loss of appetite;

+ painful and tender breasts.

6. IS MY PERIOD SUPPOSED TO HURT THIS MUCH?

It is common for women to experience pain in their lower tummy, vagina and lower back a few days before as well as during their menstrual bleeding. This is due to the walls of the uterus contracting to expel the thick layer of spongy lining from your uterus. Some women find this pain easy to manage with painkillers. If you find the pain is too difficult for you to manage, you can make an appointment with your GP who will talk to you about different medication that can make your period less painful. They may also talk about giving you hormonal contraception as this can make period less painful. If your period pain is so bad that its interfering with your ability to do daily tasks, please see a GP as this can be a sign of a medical condition such as endometriosis.

7. WHAT CAN I DO TO HELP MY PERIOD PAIN?

Pain during your period or 'menstrual bleeding' can be annoying and distressing, but most women will experience it. Depending on how much pain you are in, the following may help relieve your period pain:

+ taking some painkillers;

+ having a warm bath or shower;

+ holding a hot water bottle on your tummy;

+ eating something that makes you happy, for example chocolate;
+ doing some light and gentle exercise;
+ having a lie down or nap.

8. WHAT AGE DO PERIODS START?

Your periods will start when your body is ready during puberty usually between the ages of 8 and 16. There is nothing a woman can do to 'start' her periods. However, there are several things that can delay a woman starting her periods; for example, being underweight, doing lots of exercise or a medical condition such as Polycystic Ovary Syndrome (PCOS). If you have not started your periods by the time you are 16, please speak to your GP.

9. WHAT AGE DO PERIODS END?

A woman will continue to have periods until she goes through the menopause. This will happen usually when a woman is in her mid-40s to early 50s. Once a woman has gone through the menopause, she is unable to have biological children.

10. HOW LONG DOES MY PERIOD LAST EACH CYCLE?

The number of days you experience menstrual bleeding can vary in each cycle. On average, women experience menstrual bleeding for 4–8 days. Many things can affect the amount of time you experience menstrual bleeding such as your age and if you are on hormonal contraception.

11. MY PERIOD BLOOD IS DARKER: WHAT DOES THAT MEAN?

Darker period blood is completely normal and healthy. It is just a sign of slightly older blood. Many women experience dark brown/black blood towards the beginning or end of their period bleeding. It is also important to know that darker period blood can also be an early sign of pregnancy.

12. SOMETIMES I SEE CLUMPS IN MY PERIOD BLOOD: IS THAT NORMAL?

If you see small clumps in your period blood, these are called blood clots. They are caused by blood drying and binding together in the uterus, which are then expelled from the uterus during your menstrual bleeding. Small clumps are nothing to be worried about and are completely normal. If you see large clumps regularly, you should make an appointment with your GP as this could be a sign of an underlying medical condition.

13. HOW MUCH BLOOD DO I LOSE DURING MY PERIOD?

Although it may seem like a lot of blood at first, the average amount of blood a person loses during their period is between two and four tablespoons.

14. CAN I GET PREGNANT ON MY PERIOD?

Yes, you can get pregnant on your period. Sperm can live in the vagina and uterus for up to six days after unprotected sex. So, if you have unprotected sex towards the end of your period and then ovulate very quickly afterwards, there is the possibility the sperm can still be alive to fertilize the egg and a pregnancy can start.

15. CAN I GO SWIMMING DURING MY PERIOD?

You can absolutely go swimming on your period. It is probably better to use a tampon or menstrual cup when you go swimming. Swimming on your period is not dirty or unhygienic.

16. WHAT IS THE MENOPAUSE?

The menopause occurs when women are typically between the ages of 45 and 55. Their menstrual cycle will eventually stop, which means they stop ovulating and having periods. Once a woman goes through the menopause she can no longer conceive a child.

17. WHAT ARE IRREGULAR PERIODS?

The average length of a menstrual cycle is between 28 and 35 days long. However, some women have irregular periods, which means their menstrual cycle is a lot longer. This means that a woman may only get her period a few times each year instead of 10 to 12 times each year which is the average. Irregular periods can be common in girls who have just started puberty and then tend to regulate as the girl gets older. Irregular periods can also be a sign of the menopause in older women in their 40s and 50s.

18. WHAT CAN MAKE MY PERIOD LATE?

If you are having unprotected sex a late period could be an early sign of pregnancy. However, there are also many other factors that can delay your period, such as:

+ losing or gaining weight rapidly;

+ stress;

+ increasing the amount of exercise you are doing;

+ medical conditions such as PCOS.

19. WHAT IS PERIOD POVERTY?

Period poverty is when women and girls do not have the money to buy period products like tampons and sanitary towels. It can be very embarrassing and distressing for people. Period poverty affects people in the UK as well as other countries.

NOTE TO TEACHERS

The UK government has made it possible for all schools to have free supplies of period products for pupils that need them. Make sure your school is signed up to this initiative, so you receive free supplies and then promote this to pupils in your school. It can be very embarrassing for pupils to admit they need period products so make sure they are in an easily accessible place in the school where pupils can take the products if they need them without asking a teacher.

---

20. CAN YOU DELAY YOUR PERIOD IF YOU DO NOT WANT TO HAVE IT DURING A HOLIDAY?

If your period is due when you are going on holiday or you do not want your period during a big event, you can ask your doctor to prescribe you medication called norethisterone to delay your period. You usually need to take three norethisterone tablets a day starting four days before your period is due to start. Once you stop taking norethisterone your period will arrive a couple of days later.

SOURCES OF FURTHER INFORMATION

Betty for Schools – www.bettyeducation.com

Bloody Good Period – www.bloodygoodperiod.com

Freedom4Girls UK – www.freedom4girls.co.uk

The NHS Website – www.nhs.uk

Vagina Museum – www.vaginamuseum.co.uk

✚ CHAPTER 7
THE BODY

QUESTIONS ASKED IN THIS CHAPTER

1. *Is my penis size normal?*

2. *Are spontaneous erections normal?*

3. *What is vaginal discharge and is it normal?*

4. *Can vaginal discharge change colour?*

5. *What is the difference between a vulva and a vagina?*

6. *Is my breast size too small?*

7. *Do sexual partners care how genitals look?*

8. *Do you have to remove your pubic hair?*

9. *Is it dirty or unhygienic for girls not to remove the hair under their arms or on their legs?*

10. *Is it normal to have lumps and bumps on your penis and scrotum?*

11. *Is it normal to have lumps and bumps on your vulva?*

TEACHER GUIDANCE

It is normal to feel apprehensive and awkward when teaching or talking about the body. Our bodies are uniquely personal and all too often are associated with shame and negative feelings. It is therefore important that we as educators remove the awkwardness around talking about our bodies. The shame around saying the correct names for our body parts like 'vulva', 'vagina' and 'penis' is still present among adults and pupils. By using these correct names when teaching about the body you are not only destigmatising the shame and embarrassment around these body parts, but you are also empowering pupils and promoting a respect for their bodies. It is also important to know the correct names for body parts in case pupils ever need to see a medical professional or for any safeguarding reasons.

Young people are increasingly showing signs of disliking their bodies and seeking medical intervention to obtain 'the perfect body'. This is particularly prevalent among young girls who are reportedly seeking cosmetic surgery on their labia and vulva because they think the way their vulva looks is 'disgusting' or 'ugly'. One could argue that this new desire to have a 'perfect vulva' stems from pornography with porn performers showcasing a very specific type of body and by extension a certain type of vulva. However, I believe this also stems from a lack of representation and exposure to different images of genitals in RSE. The way to tackle this is to show different diagrams or drawings of vulvas and penises when talking about reproductive anatomy. This will then reinforce to pupils that all genitals look different and that is completely healthy.

QUESTIONS

1. IS MY PENIS SIZE NORMAL?

Yes. Penises come in all shapes and sizes. Some have a slight bend to the left or right. Some bend upward or downwards. Everyone is different. The important thing to remember is that your penis is completely normal and healthy.

2. ARE SPONTANEOUS ERECTIONS NORMAL?

Spontaneous erections are completely normal and may happen a lot during puberty. Some boys may experience many and some boys won't get any spontaneous erections at all. Although you may find them embarrassing, they are completely natural and healthy and all part of your body changing from a child to an adult.

3. WHAT IS VAGINAL DISCHARGE AND IS IT NORMAL?

Vaginal discharge is a fluid that leaks out of the vagina. It is normal and healthy for girls and women to experience vaginal discharge daily. Girls will start to get vaginal discharge during puberty and this can often be a sign that your period may be about to start. Vaginal discharge is your vagina's way of cleaning itself and protects the vagina from infections. Some girls worry about the amount of vaginal discharge they get and believe it is dirty. This is not true, and you should not worry. Some girls wear very thin panty liners in their underwear to stop the vaginal discharge from staining their underwear.

4. CAN VAGINAL DISCHARGE CHANGE COLOUR?

Vaginal discharge can often change colour and consistency. It can change from watery and clear to thick with a yellow tinge during your menstrual cycle. If your vaginal discharge is green or very yellow this could be the sign of a bacterial infection or an STI. If your vaginal discharge is brown this is probably a sign that your period is about to start as it means your vaginal discharge has mixed with blood. Vaginal discharge should not itch, burn, cause redness or look like cottage cheese in consistency. If you have any of these symptoms it is important to see your GP as this could be a sign of infection.

5. WHAT IS THE DIFFERENCE BETWEEN A VULVA AND A VAGINA?

The vulva is the name of the external part of a woman's genitals. The vulva includes the labia minora, labia majora, clitoris, vaginal opening and urethra opening. The vagina is the name of the internal canal that stretches from the vaginal opening to the cervix at the entrance of the uterus.

6. IS MY BREAST SIZE TOO SMALL?

During puberty every girl's breasts will develop at different rates. Remember a girl's body doesn't fully stop growing until they are around 18 or 19. Breasts come in all shapes and sizes and that's completely normal. Some girls with smaller breasts can wear special bras that make their breasts appear larger. It is important for you to feel happy with your breast size. If you are worried or upset about your breast size, then talk to your GP.

7. DO SEXUAL PARTNERS CARE HOW GENITALS LOOK?

Some people have ideas and expect a person's genitals to look a certain way. There are many reasons for this including what they have seen in films or TV, what they have seen in pornography or what they have heard from friends. The important thing to remember is that no sexual partner should force you to change the appearance of your genitals. If you are happy with the way your genitals look then that is all that matters, and your sexual partner should respect that.

8. DO YOU HAVE TO REMOVE YOUR PUBIC HAIR?

Removing your pubic hair is entirely your own choice. No one should ever force you to remove your pubic hair if you do not want to. You also should not feel you have to remove your pubic hair because your friends do it or it's what you've heard in the media.

9. IS IT DIRTY OR UNHYGIENIC FOR GIRLS NOT TO REMOVE THE HAIR UNDER THEIR ARMS OR ON THEIR LEGS?

You may have heard some people talking about leg hair, pubic hair and underarm hair as 'dirty' or 'gross'; this is false. Hair on your body acts as a barrier to stop bacteria from getting to your skin and is not dirty or unhygienic at all. Some people like to remove their hair, but this is a personal choice. You do not need to remove your body hair if you do not want to.

10. IS IT NORMAL TO HAVE LUMPS AND BUMPS ON YOUR PENIS AND SCROTUM?

It is common during puberty to see little skin-coloured lumps on the shaft of your penis. These are likely to be visible hair folicles protruding through the skin and are harmless. You can also get skin cysts on your penis or scrotum, which are nothing to worry about. If you have had unprotected sex and you notice new lumps on your penis it could be a sign of an STI like herpes or genital warts. The best thing to do if you are ever concerned about lumps on your penis or scrotum is to make an appointment with your GP for advice. Never try to remove a lump on your penis yourself.

11. IS IT NORMAL TO HAVE LUMPS AND BUMPS ON YOUR VULVA?

If you find lumps on your vulva this could be due to a number of things. Small red lumps can be due to a shaving rash and will go away in a few days. Skin-coloured hard lumps could be a cyst. While these may look scary they are nothing to worry about and can often be caused by ingrown hairs or friction between the vulva and tight underwear. If you have had unprotected sex and you notice new lumps on your vulva, this could be a sign of an STI like herpes or genital warts. The best thing to do if you are ever concerned about lumps on your vulva is to make an appointment with your GP for advice. Never try to remove a lump on your vulva yourself.

SOURCES OF FURTHER INFORMATION

Brook – www.brook.org.uk

Childline – www.childline.org.uk

The NHS Website – www.nhs.uk

NSPCC – www.nspcc.org.uk

The Mix – www.themix.org.uk

✚ CHAPTER 8
GENDER

QUESTIONS ASKED IN THIS CHAPTER

1. *What does trans/transgender mean?*
2. *What does non-binary mean?*
3. *What does intersex mean?*
4. *What does transitioning mean?*
5. *What does transexual mean?*
6. *What does transvestite mean?*
7. *What is tucking?*
8. *What is binding?*
9. *Am I transgender if I cross-dress?*
10. *What does gender neutral mean?*
11. *What does gender fluid mean?*
12. *What does gender dysphoria mean?*
13. *Why is it important to call someone by the correct personal pronouns?*
14. *Can people who change gender get a new birth certificate and passport?*
15. *What is the difference between sex and gender?*

TEACHER GUIDANCE

Gender, like sexuality, is still seen as a very complex issue. Some teachers and pupils may struggle to understand different gender identities and transgender issues. In order to build an inclusive school for pupils who identify as transgender, a whole school approach needs to be taken. This means that transgender issues and diversity should be discussed and celebrated outside the classroom. This can be done by having displays around the school about inspirational transgender people who can be role models to pupils or by holding transgender awareness assemblies.

As a school you have a duty to make RSE trans-inclusive. This means not just talking about transgender issues and diversity in its own separate topic but also including it in other RSE topics such as puberty. Puberty can be a very difficult time for pupils who do not identify as the same gender they were assigned at birth. It is therefore important that trans puberty is discussed during puberty sessions. It is also a good idea (as you may not know how many pupils identify as transgender in your class) not to use gendered words when talking about changes during puberty. For example, instead of using the phrase *here are some of the changes boys go through during puberty* you could say *here are some of the changes people with penises go through during puberty*. Not only does this make puberty lessons more inclusive for pupils who may identify as transgender, but it also provides the opportunity for further discussions with pupils on gender and what gender means to different people.

QUESTIONS

1. WHAT DOES TRANS/TRANSGENDER MEAN?

Transgender is the general term that can be used to identify anyone whose gender does not match their biological sex they were assigned at birth.

2. WHAT DOES NON-BINARY MEAN?

Non-binary is the general term that can be used to describe people who do not identity within the stereotypical gender binary of male or female. Non-binary people can fluctuate between the two genders or not identify as any gender.

3. WHAT DOES INTERSEX MEAN?

Intersex is a term used to describe someone who has the biological characteristics of both male and female. This could mean they have both male and female reproductive organs or chromosomes. In the past intersex people were called hermaphrodites. This is now seen as derogatory and offensive. Intersex people may choose to live as male, female or non-binary.

4. WHAT DOES TRANSITIONING MEAN?

Transitioning is the name given to the process in which a person takes steps to live as the gender they identify as. People can transition in different ways: medically, which means undergoing hormone therapy or gender affirmation surgery; legally, where people change their gender on legal documents such as their passports and birth certificates; or socially, where people specify their preferred pronouns or name they would like to be known as.

5. WHAT DOES TRANSEXUAL MEAN?

Transexual was a term used to describe transgender people in the past. Many people see this as an outdated term and prefer to use the word transgender.

6. WHAT DOES TRANSVESTITE MEAN?

Transvestite is an outdated term for people who dress and act in the opposite gender to which they were assigned at birth. 'Cross-dressing' is the preferred term to describe this now.

7. WHAT IS TUCKING?

Tucking is the term given to people who hide their penis and testicles so they cannot be seen through clothing. Transgender people who were assigned male at birth may do this in order to look female or for their own personal comfort. Tucking can also be used by people who cross-dress as women.

8. WHAT IS BINDING?

Binding is the term given to wrapping your breasts with tight material to reduce the appearance of them. Transgender people who were assigned female at birth may do this in order to look male or for their own comfort. Not all transgender people take part in binding.

9. AM I TRANSGENDER IF I CROSS-DRESS?

Cross-dressing does not have anything to do with your gender identity. Cross-dressing is a form of gender expression and sometimes a part of entertainment, for example, drag or stand-up comedy. Some people who identify as transgender or non-binary may choose to cross-dress but it should never be assumed that everyone who cross-dresses identifies as transgender/non-binary.

10. WHAT DOES GENDER NEUTRAL MEAN?

Gender neutral means to not class someone/something as specifically masculine or feminine. If someone identifies themselves as gender neutral that means they do not associate themselves with a specific gender. While if an object or facility is gender neutral, for example, gender-neutral toilets, this means that there are no restrictions on who can use it as it is open to all genders.

11. WHAT DOES GENDER FLUID MEAN?

Gender fluid is the term given to describe someone's gender identity that is not fixed but can change over time. If someone identifies as gender fluid this can mean that sometimes they can identity more with one gender than the other while other times not identify as any gender at all.

12. WHAT DOES GENDER DYSPHORIA MEAN?

Gender dysphoria is the term given to the feeling of distress or discomfort when someone does not identify with the biological sex they were assigned at birth. Gender dysphoria can sometimes lead to mental health issues such as anxiety, depression and suicidal thoughts. It is therefore extremely important to take gender dysphoria seriously and support people who are experiencing it.

13. WHY IS IT IMPORTANT TO CALL SOMEONE BY THE CORRECT PERSONAL PRONOUNS?

It is extremely important to call someone by their preferred personal pronouns. This could be 'he/him', 'she/her', 'they/them', 'ze/sir'. If you do not call someone by their correct personal pronouns, this can be very upsetting and damaging to that person's mental health and self-esteem as you are denying that person their gender identity. If you are unsure of someone's preferred personal pronouns, it is always best to ask them. Never assume a person's personal pronouns based on their outward gender expression.

14. CAN PEOPLE WHO CHANGE GENDER GET A NEW BIRTH CERTIFICATE AND PASSPORT?

People who identify as transgender can legally change their gender on their birth certificate by applying for a legal document called a gender recognition certificate. You must be 18 or over to apply for this. Not all people who identify as transgender want a gender recognition certificate but some people feel this is an important part of their transitioning process.

15. WHAT IS THE DIFFERENCE BETWEEN SEX AND GENDER?

Your biological sex is to do with your reproductive characteristics you were born with; for example, whether you have male, female or intersex genitals and your chromosomes. Your gender is a socially constructed idea about whether you should behave more masculine or feminine depending on which biological sex you were assigned at birth.

SOURCES OF FURTHER INFORMATION

Brook – www.brook.org.uk

Childine – www.childline.org.uk

Galop – www.galop.org.uk

Stonewall – www.stonewall.org.uk

Trans Unite – www.transunite.co.uk

✚ CHAPTER 9
SEXUALITY

QUESTIONS ASKED IN THIS CHAPTER

1. *I have heard someone say they are queer: isn't that offensive?*

2. *What does asexual mean?*

3. *Isn't bisexual and pansexual the same thing?*

4. *Is it okay to not feel any sexual feelings for anyone?*

5. *Can you tell if someone is gay by looking at them?*

6. *When do you know your sexuality?*

7. *What does LGBTQ+ mean?*

8. *When is the right time to come out/how should I come out?*

9. *What if my friends/family do not accept my sexuality?*

10. *My faith/culture does not accept my sexuality: what should I do?*

11. *Why do some people not accept bisexuality as a real sexuality?*

12. *I am under 18 and I think I am LGBTQ+. Do I legally have to disclose my sexuality to my parents/guardians?*

13. *What does 'questioning' mean?*

14. *What does cisgender mean?*

15. *What does 'ally' mean?*

71

TEACHER GUIDANCE

Sexuality is a topic that is both complex and personal. In the past 50 years, there have been great leaps in acceptance and understanding towards sexuality and the LGBTQ+ community. Unfortunately, you still get some people who disagree with any sexuality that is not heteronormative, be that for either cultural or religious reasons. It is your role as the educator to foster an inclusive and open atmosphere to LGBTQ+ issues within the classroom. In previous years RSE has been very heteronormatively focused, for example, only talking about safe sex practices between a man and a woman or talking about healthy and unhealthy relationship scenarios between a heterosexual man and woman. Such practices in the classroom are alienating to the pupils who do not identify as heterosexual and furthermore deny these pupils valuable information to practise safe and healthy relationships.

Many educators will dedicate an entire lesson to learning about LGBTQ+ relationships, diversity and tolerance. While beneficial, sometimes the best way to tackle heteronormative values within RSE and promote openness and understanding is not to separate LGBTQ+ issues into separate lessons but to integrate it into main topic lessons alongside talking about heterosexual relationships. An example of how you can do this is to always use the word 'partner' and not 'boyfriend/girlfriend' when talking about potential romantic and sexual relationships. When talking about relationship scenarios during discussions always give the characters in the scenario gender-neutral names like Charlie, Jamie, Jo, Jordan, etc. This allows pupils to not make assumptions about the character's sexuality and gender. Finally, when talking about sexual activity, do not solely focus on heteronormative penis in vagina penetrative sex, but also discuss anal sex, oral sex and sexual touching.

As an educator you should be alert to any homophobic or biphobia remarks that a pupil may make during an RSE lesson. Phrases like 'that is so gay' or 'no homo' are both examples of homophobic remarks. While these phrases may have passed into common and frequent use by pupils, you still have a duty as an educator to challenge these remarks. These phrases associate the word 'gay' with being a negative thing and by extension give LGBTQ+ relationships negative connotations. While most of the time these phrases are said by pupils without thinking and stem from ignorance rather than intolerance, it is important to not let this behaviour go unchallenged. By allowing pupils use these phrases in commonplace language, it can escalate into more serious homophobic behaviour.

QUESTIONS

1. I HAVE HEARD SOMEONE SAY THEY ARE QUEER: ISN'T THAT OFFENSIVE?

If you are calling someone queer as a way of insulting them, that is offensive. However, a lot of LGBTQ+ people have now reclaimed the meaning of the word queer to mean a positive thing. Queer is now seen as an umbrella term for anyone who is not exclusively heterosexual.

2. WHAT DOES ASEXUAL MEAN?

A person who identifies as asexual does not experience any sexual attraction to others. However, some people who identify as asexual may experience romantic feelings for other people and have romantic relationships. People who identify as asexual may sometimes call themselves 'Ace'.

3. ISN'T BISEXUAL AND PANSEXUAL THE SAME THING?

Bisexual means to be attracted to the same gender as yourself as well as other genders. Pansexual means to be attracted to all genders. While both these sexualities seem to be similar, the key difference is that for pansexual people, a person's gender plays no role in whether they are sexually/romantically attractive. You might say that people who identify as pansexual are 'gender blind', while people who identify as bisexual may consider a person's gender as part of what makes them sexually/romantically attractive.

4. IS IT OKAY TO NOT FEEL ANY SEXUAL FEELINGS FOR ANYONE?

It is completely normal to not feel any sexual attraction to anyone during puberty. These feelings may develop later or not at all.

5. CAN YOU TELL IF SOMEONE IS GAY BY LOOKING AT THEM?

No. The way people express themselves through appearance can be completely unrelated to their sexuality. You should never assume anyone's sexuality or gender based on their appearance.

6. WHEN DO YOU KNOW YOUR SEXUALITY?

Sexuality is a very complex thing, but it is also very fluid and can actually change during our lives. During puberty you may start to develop feelings for people of the opposite biological sex or same biological sex as you. This is completely normal.

Some people know their sexuality quite early on in their lives and others take longer. Whatever your sexuality is, you must remember that it is your sexuality that is private and personal to you. You should never feel forced to reveal your sexuality or present a sexuality that is different to your own.

If you feel that life would become dangerous for you if your sexuality was revealed, please seek help and advice. There are lots of great LGBTQ+ charities who can help, such as Stonewall.

7. WHAT DOES LGBTQ+ MEAN?

LGBTQ+ stands for lesbian, gay, bisexual, transgender and queer/questioning. The plus symbol signifies all other possible non-heterosexual sexualities as a way of being inclusive.

8. WHEN IS THE RIGHT TIME TO COME OUT/ HOW SHOULD I COME OUT?

You should be the one to decide when/how you come out about your sexuality. There is no right time to come out about your sexuality and you should only start to tell people when you feel comfortable doing so.

9. WHAT IF MY FRIENDS/FAMILY DO NOT ACCEPT MY SEXUALITY?

If you choose to tell your friends and family about your sexuality, there is the possibility that they may not accept your sexuality. This could be because your sexuality has come as a shock to them. Give them time to think and process what you have told them, and this could help them understand and accept your sexuality. If your friends and family still do not accept your sexuality after having time to process it, then ultimately there may be nothing you can do. It is important to remember that even if your friends and family do not accept your sexuality, your sexuality is still valid and not wrong.

10. MY FAITH/CULTURE DOES NOT ACCEPT MY SEXUALITY: WHAT SHOULD I DO?

If you have been raised in a faith or culture that does not accept your sexuality, there is no need to disclose your sexuality to members of your community. Your sexuality is private and personal to you, especially if you feel like disclosing your sexuality would put you in personal danger from your community. There are many LGBTQ+ groups within religions that can support you.

11. WHY DO SOME PEOPLE NOT ACCEPT BISEXUALITY AS A REAL SEXUALITY?

Some people feel that bisexuality is not a real sexuality and may use biphobic phrases such as 'Bisexual people cannot make up their mind' or 'Bisexuals are just greedy'. This thinking is very prejudiced and intolerant. It can also be very harmful to people who identify as bisexual as it makes them feel that their sexuality is not valid and can cause mental health issues.

12. I AM UNDER 18 AND I THINK I AM LGBTQ+. DO I LEGALLY HAVE TO DISCLOSE MY SEXUALITY TO MY PARENTS/GUARDIANS?

Your sexuality is private and intimate to you. Even if you are under 18 you are not obligated legally or morally to tell anyone your sexuality if you do not feel comfortable doing so.

13. WHAT DOES 'QUESTIONING' MEAN?

If someone describes themselves as questioning, it can mean they are curious or exploring a part of their sexuality or gender.

14. WHAT DOES CISGENDER MEAN?

Cisgender is the term given to anyone whose gender identity matches the biological sex they were assigned at birth.

15. WHAT DOES 'ALLY' MEAN?

An ally is a person who identifies as heterosexual or cisgender who supports LGBTQ+ relationships and equality.

SOURCES OF FURTHER INFORMATION

Brook – www.brook.org.uk

LGBT Foundation – www.lgbt.foundation

Metro Charity – www.metro.org.uk

Stonewall – www.stonewall.co.uk

Switchboard LGBT – www.stwichboard.lgbt

✚ CHAPTER 10
PREGNANCY CHOICES

QUESTIONS ASKED IN THIS CHAPTER

1. *What is abortion?*

2. *Is abortion the same as miscarriage?*

3. *What are the different types of abortions?*

4. *Is abortion murder? What do you think about abortion?*

5. *How do you get an abortion?*

6. *Do you have to tell your parents if you want an abortion?*

7. *Should I tell my partner if I am thinking of getting an abortion?*

8. *Can my partner legally stop me from getting an abortion?*

9. *Up to how many weeks pregnant can you get an abortion?*

10. *Will I and my partner be reported to the police by a medical professional if I am under 16 and I am trying to get an abortion?*

11. *Can I get an abortion from my GP?*

12. *How does adoption work?*

13. *Can you still go to sixth form or university if you are pregnant?*

14. *What age is the right time to become a parent?*

15. *Why can some people not have biological children?*

16. *What is IVF?*

TEACHER GUIDANCE

Pregnancy choices can be a sensitive topic for both staff and pupils. Your religion, faith or culture may make you feel conflicted about teaching pupils about abortion. While this may be uncomfortable for you, it is important to remember that you are not being asked to give your personal opinion on abortion but teach facts you are required to teach by the Department for Education. If you are truly uncomfortable about teaching abortion or do not wish to teach it due to distressing personal experiences, please talk to your line manager or the Head of Well-being/PSHE at your school.

QUESTIONS

1. WHAT IS ABORTION?

An abortion is a safe medical procedure that ends a pregnancy. You might sometimes hear the word 'termination' instead of abortion, but it means the same thing.

2. IS ABORTION THE SAME AS MISCARRIAGE?

A miscarriage is sometimes called a 'spontaneous abortion', so it can be easy to think they are both similar. A miscarriage is when the foetus or embryo dies of natural causes in the uterus. The uterus will then expel the pregnancy itself or sometimes medical help is needed to remove the dead foetus or embryo. An abortion is when a woman receives a medical procedure to end her pregnancy.

3. WHAT ARE THE DIFFERENT TYPES OF ABORTIONS?

There are three different methods of abortion. The method of abortion used depends on how many weeks into your pregnancy you are.

+ **Medical abortion** (up to ten weeks): This involves taking two medicines. The first is Mifepristone, which ends the pregnancy by stopping the foetus develop, and the second is Misoprostol, which expels the pregnancy through cramping and bleeding. Most women expel the pregnancy within four hours, but it can sometimes take longer. Women may experience bleeding like the bleeding you would get with a period for around 1–2 weeks after this type of abortion.

+ **Vacuum or suction method** (up to 15 weeks): A woman is given anaesthetic, but she can choose whether she wants to be awake or asleep. A narrow tube is passed through the cervix at the top of the vagina and into the uterus. The procedure is very quick and there is no scarring caused. Women may experience bleeding like their period for a week afterwards.

+ **Surgical dilation and evacuation** (15 to 24 weeks): This is a minor operation done under general anaesthetic while the woman is asleep. The cervix at the entrance of the uterus will be gently stretched and the pregnancy will be removed using a suction tube and surgical instruments. Most women go home the same day, but some may need to stay overnight in hospital. Afterwards patients may experience bleeding for up to three weeks.

4. IS ABORTION MURDER? WHAT DO YOU THINK ABOUT ABORTION?

We are not here to discuss my personal opinions towards abortion. I am here to make sure you all understand what it is and the facts about it. There are many different beliefs and feelings about abortion but the appropriate time to discuss them would be in a Religious Education or Citizenship lesson.

5. HOW DO YOU GET AN ABORTION?

If you decide you want an abortion, the first step would be to see your GP or go to a sexual health clinic. They can give you more information about the abortion process and refer to a specialist service that carries out abortions. You will not need to pay for the abortion or any medical appointments as these are all free on the NHS.

6. DO YOU HAVE TO TELL YOUR PARENTS IF YOU WANT AN ABORTION?

If a young person fully understands the choices they are making and it is their own choice to have an abortion, a doctor can arrange an abortion without your parents' knowledge or involvement. This includes if the person seeking an abortion is under 16. No one will pressure you to tell your parents about your abortion and you do not have to tell them if you do not want to. If you do not tell your parents about your abortion your doctor will advise you to tell someone who is over 16 for support.

7. SHOULD I TELL MY PARTNER IF I AM THINKING OF GETTING AN ABORTION?

You do not have to tell anyone if you do not want to, that you are thinking of getting an abortion. You may want to tell your partner so they can support you. Ultimately, you must be the one who decides whether you should have an abortion.

8. CAN MY PARTNER LEGALLY STOP ME FROM GETTING AN ABORTION?

Your partner cannot legally stop you from getting an abortion. In the UK, all the legal rights are owned by the woman who is pregnant to decide what she wants to do about her pregnancy.

9. UP TO HOW MANY WEEKS PREGNANT CAN YOU GET AN ABORTION?

Most abortions in the UK are performed earlier than 12 weeks. Legally, a woman can access an abortion any time before she is 24 weeks' pregnant. An abortion will only be carried out after 24 weeks in exceptional circumstances, such as when the mother's life would be put at risk if she continues with the pregnancy to full term.

10. WILL I AND MY PARTNER BE REPORTED TO THE POLICE BY A MEDICAL PROFESSIONAL IF I AM UNDER 16 AND I AM TRYING TO GET AN ABORTION?

Although the age of consent in the UK is 16, the purpose of the law is to protect not to prosecute young people. If two people under the age of 16 have had consensual sex it is classed as illegal sex, but it is highly unlikely a medical professional would report this to the police. Neither a man nor a woman's age will affect their rights to access an abortion.

11. CAN I GET AN ABORTION FROM MY GP?

No, a GP cannot perform an abortion. However, you can make an appointment with your GP to find out more about abortion. Your GP can also refer you to a specialist service that provides abortions.

12. HOW DOES ADOPTION WORK?

If you have decided you want your child to be adopted, you will need to contact a social worker to get advice and make sure adoption is the right decision for you. You can make contact with a social worker through an adoption charity or through social services in your local area. Once you are certain about adoption, a social worker will sort out the adoption process for you. They will need to know some personal information about you and your family. This is for your child's adoptive parents to be aware of your child's medical history. When your baby is born a social worker will take the baby and place it with temporary foster parents or its adoptive parents. Once an adoption has been made legal through the courts you will have no legal relationship or rights with your baby.

13. CAN YOU STILL GO TO SIXTH FORM OR UNIVERSITY IF YOU ARE PREGNANT?

You can still go to sixth form or university if you are pregnant. You should tell your sixth form or university that you are pregnant as they may have services in place that can assist you with your studying. Studying while pregnant can be difficult and tiring so you may want to consider taking a year's gap or break from your studies during your pregnancy.

14. WHAT AGE IS THE RIGHT TIME TO BECOME A PARENT?

There is never a 'right' age to become a parent. Some parents feel ready to have a baby when they are in their teens, while others wait until they are in their 30s or 40s. It is important to consider that even though your body may be ready to have a baby, you may not be ready to have a baby mentally or financially. You should consider your support network and if you have friends and family who can help you with your child if you are struggling.

15. WHY CAN SOME PEOPLE NOT HAVE BIOLOGICAL CHILDREN?

Some people have problems conceiving a child. This is called infertility. There are many things that can cause infertility such as:

+ a woman's fallopian tubes being blocked so an egg cannot travel to the uterus;

+ a woman does not release eggs regularly (irregular menstrual cycles);

+ a lining of a woman's uterus may not be thick enough for an egg to implant;

+ a man has a low sperm count;

+ a man's sperm has low mobility, which means the sperm are likely to die before reaching an egg.

Sometimes these issues can be fixed with medical procedures and other times they cannot. Infertility issues can be very stressful and upsetting for people who are trying to have a baby.

16. WHAT IS IVF?

IVF stands for 'in vitro fertilisation' and can be a solution to parents who are struggling to conceive a baby biologically. During IVF an egg is removed by a medical professional from a woman's ovary and fertilised with sperm in a laboratory. The fertilised egg, which is called an embryo, is then returned to the woman's womb to grow and develop.

SOURCES OF FURTHER INFORMATION

BPAS: British Pregnancy Advisory Service – www.bpas.org

Brook – www.brook.org.uk

Marie Stopes Clinics – www.msichoices.org.uk

Plan International UK – www.plan-uk.org

Women's Aid – www.womensaid.org.uk

✚ CHAPTER 11
PORNOGRAPHY

QUESTIONS ASKED IN THIS CHAPTER

1. *What is pornography?*

2. *How old do you have to be to watch pornography?*

3. *Is it illegal for two 17 year-olds to watch pornography together?*

4. *What do I do if I have been shown/accidently watch pornography?*

5. *If my partner is 18 and I am 16, is it okay to watch pornography because one of us is an adult?*

6. *Is it bad to watch pornography if you are an adult?*

7. *Is it bad that I am watching pornography because I want to find out about sex?*

8. *What is revenge porn?*

9. *Is it wrong for my partner and I to make a sex tape if we are both 18?*

10. *What happens if I accidentally see images or videos of someone under 18 on a porn site?*

11. *If I watch porn without my partner knowing, does this count as cheating?*

12. *How do you know if you are watching too much porn?*

TEACHER GUIDANCE

Today pornographic images and videos are more readily available and accessible than they have ever been before. A lot of pornographic content is also free via the internet. Due to this, pupils are being exposed to pornography at an younger age than previous generations. Findings from some studies suggest that by the age of 12 many children would have been exposed to some sort of pornography. While this may be shocking to most adults, the way to combat this young exposure to pornography is to make sure pupils receive a thorough education about pornography within RSE. The way to deliver this education is to have open, honest and non-judgemental conversations with pupils.

In order to facilitate a thorough education on pornography, it is important to know the reasons why pupils might be watching pornography. By knowing the exact reasons, you are more likely to relate to pupils and build a classroom atmosphere that is open and honest. There are many reasons why a pupil may have seen pornography at a younger age, but the most common reasons are as follows.

1. They have been shown by friends/want to appear rebellious in front of their friends.

2. They are curious about sex and want to find out more.

3. They are trying to work out their sexuality.

4. They have been shown by an older partner.

5. They are using it as a tool to stimulate themselves sexually during masturbation.

6. They have been exposed to it as a grooming and child sexual exploitation (CSE) tactic.

If a pupil has seen pornography because of reasons one or five, it is important to remind them about the laws surrounding viewing pornography. Emphasise that the laws around under 18s viewing pornography are there to protect and not to punish pupils. Reasons two and three for watching pornography are probably the most understandable reasons. Again, it is important to emphasise the laws around pornography but also discuss how pornography often shows unrealistic depictions of sexual acts. It also rarely shows important concepts like consent negotiation and condom/contraception use.

QUESTIONS

1. WHAT IS PORNOGRAPHY?

Pornography is graphic images or videos of sexual acts or genitals intended to arouse (turn on) the person viewing/watching them.

2. HOW OLD DO YOU HAVE TO BE TO WATCH PORNOGRAPHY?

In the UK you must be 18 before you watch pornography.

3. IS IT ILLEGAL FOR TWO 17 YEAR-OLDS TO WATCH PORNOGRAPHY TOGETHER?

Even if you both want to watch pornography the legal age for watching pornography is 18. Therefore, two 17 year-olds watching porn together is illegal.

4. WHAT DO I DO IF I HAVE BEEN SHOWN/ ACCIDENTLY WATCH PORNOGRAPHY?

If you have been shown pornography without your consent or accidently seen it online and it has upset or distressed you, you should talk to an adult that you trust. They will not be upset or judge you. It is important for your mental health that you talk to someone about what you have seen. You can also find support from various online websites such as Brook.org.uk and CEOP.org.uk (see 'Sources of further information' at the end of this chapter).

5. IF MY PARTNER IS 18 AND I AM 16, IS IT OKAY TO WATCH PORNOGRAPHY BECAUSE ONE OF US IS AN ADULT?

Even if your partner is 18, the law is there to protect under 18s which means it would still be illegal for an 18 and a 16 year-old to watch pornography together. There would also be serious legal consequences for the 18 year-old as it is against the law for any adult to show pornography to someone under the age of 18 as this is classed as indirect sexual abuse.

6. IS IT BAD TO WATCH PORNOGRAPHY IF YOU ARE AN ADULT?

If you are 18 or over, it is your choice whether you want to watch pornography or not. There are some types of pornography that are illegal to watch even as an adult. This includes pornography showing:

+ people under the age of 18;

+ sex with animals (bestiality);

+ sex with dead people (necrophilia);

+ sex where serious bodily harm is caused;

+ rape.

7. IS IT BAD THAT I AM WATCHING PORNOGRAPHY BECAUSE I WANT TO FIND OUT ABOUT SEX?

It is completely natural and normal to be curious about sex. However, pornography (even though it may seem very realistic) does not always accurately portray what sex is like. Pornography has been created with the intention to excite and arouse (turn on) people. Due to this, a lot of aspects of pornography may have been exaggerated. If you want to find out about sex, there are lots of books appropriate for your age you can read. There are also lots of sexual health websites specifically for children and teenagers that talk about sex.

NOTE TO TEACHERS

It is a great idea to have a few books on sex and relationships available in the school library for pupils to browse whenever they want. You may also have a school nurse who regularly hosts information drop-in sessions for pupils. If you have these resources available in your school, you can remind your pupils of this during RSE lessons.

---

8. WHAT IS REVENGE PORN?

Revenge porn is when an explicit picture or video is shown to the public without the consent of the people who appear in the image or video. An example of this is if two people who were in a sexual relationship with each other made a video of them having sex and then broke up. Then one person released the video to the public, by sharing it online or with their group of friends without their ex-partner's consent. This would be revenge porn. Revenge porn is wrong at any age and can have serious legal consequences for people who take part in it. This can include a prison sentence of up to two years. If the person featured in the videos or pictures of revenge porn is under 18, this can have even more serious consequences as this is then classed as distributing indecent images/videos of a child.

9. IS IT WRONG FOR MY PARTNER AND I TO MAKE A SEX TAPE IF WE ARE BOTH 18?

If you and your partner are both over the age of 18 and are both consenting it is legal to make a sex tape if you want to. Even though it is legal, you might want to consider some of the long-term consequences of making a sex tape if your sex tape is shared with people you did not intend it to be shared with.

10. WHAT HAPPENS IF I ACCIDENTALLY SEE IMAGES OR VIDEOS OF SOMEONE UNDER 18 ON A PORN SITE?

If you see images or videos of someone under 18 on a porn site, you should report it immediately to the site administrator of that website. You should also report it to CEOP, the organisation for child protection on the internet. If you are under 18 yourself, you won't get into trouble for reporting pornography that has under 18 year-olds in it.

11. IF I WATCH PORN WITHOUT MY PARTNER KNOWING, DOES THIS COUNT AS CHEATING?

This question does not have a right or wrong answer. Some partners may see this as cheating and other partners may be completely fine with their partner watching pornography. The best thing to do is communicate with your partner and see what they feel about it. If your partner does not feel comfortable with you watching pornography and it upsets them, but you would still like to watch pornography, you will need to have further discussions with your partner about relationship boundaries.

12. HOW DO YOU KNOW IF YOU ARE WATCHING TOO MUCH PORN?

When it comes to watching pornography, everyone is different. Some people may only watch it occasionally while others may watch it several times a week. If you feel that you cannot go a day without watching pornography or watching pornography is all you think about then you may have developed a porn addiction. There are several organisations that can help with this (see Sources of further information below). If the amount of pornography you are watching is worrying you, you may want to tell an adult you trust so they can support and help you.

SOURCES OF FURTHER INFORMATION

Brook – www.brook.org.uk

CEOP (Child Exploitation and Online Protection) – www.ceop.police.uk/safety-centre/

Childline – www.childline.org.uk

Disrespect Nobody – www.disrespectnobody.co.uk

NSPCC – www.nspcc.org.uk

Bish Training – https://bishtraining.com/planet-porn

✚ CHAPTER 12
SEXTING

QUESTIONS ASKED IN THIS CHAPTER

1. *What is sexting?*

2. *Why do people sext?*

3. *Can you send a naked picture to your partner if you are 17 and in a relationship?*

4. *What happens if you have a nude image of an under 18 on your phone?*

5. *Is it okay if I take a naked picture of myself if I am under 18 and not send it to anyone?*

6. *Can you go to prison if you have a nude picture on your phone?*

7. *What should I do if I receive a naked picture?*

8. *What should I do if a nude picture of me has been shared around?*

9. *What should I do if someone is pressuring me to send a nude picture?*

TEACHER GUIDANCE

In recent years, due to the widespread use of smartphones among under 18s, there has been a growing concern over the number of pupils who are engaging in sexting. Similar to when teaching about pornography, it is important that teachers do not shame, judge or scaremonger pupils when teaching about sexting. It is also important to understand the reasons why young people engage in sexting in order to educate them properly of the consequences. The reasons why pupils may engage in sexting are:

1. to feel intimate and close to someone in a relationship;

2. to feel grown up and imitate adult behaviour;

3. they are being pressured or blackmailed into sexting;

4. to receive a boost to their self-esteem.

Reason one is easy to understand as most adults will engage in sexting for this reason, particularly if the relationship is long distance. Sexting between two people also builds trust and establishes a close bond. However, it is important to remind pupils about the laws surrounding sexting if they are under 18. You can also educate pupils about other ways they can build intimacy and bond in a relationship without engaging in sexting. Reason two again is understandable. During adolescence pupils want to push boundaries and try new things and they may consider trying sexting. A way to counter this thinking in pupils is to explain that part of growing up and maturing is also being aware of the legal consequences of sexting as well as the long-term social consequences. For example, once you have sent a naked picture online this could be found several years later by potential employers.

Pupils may also feel pressured into sexting by their peers or by a partner. It is important to educate pupils that this is never okay. It can be difficult for pupils to say no to sexting when they are being bullied by others. There are a lot of websites that pupils can visit for help on this such as the Zipit app (created by Childline) that can be used to send funny comebacks to someone who is pressuring them to send naked images.

QUESTIONS

1. WHAT IS SEXTING?

Sexting is the term for sending or receiving sexually explicit images, videos or messages, usually through a mobile phone.

2. WHY DO PEOPLE SEXT?

People take part in sexting for many different reasons such as:

+ they feel bored and think it is a fun thing to do;

+ they want someone to compliment them on how they look;

+ to build trust in a relationship;

+ to feel close to someone in a relationship;

+ to maintain intimacy with someone in a long-distance relationship;

+ they are being pressured into sexting by friends or a partner.

It is important to remember that it is illegal to take part in sexting if you are under the age of 18. When you are 18, it is your own personal choice whether you want to take part in sexting or not.

3. CAN YOU SEND A NAKED PICTURE TO YOUR PARTNER IF YOU ARE 17 AND IN A RELATIONSHIP?

Even though you are over the age of consent, at 17 you are still classed as a child by UK law. Therefore, any naked pictures of a 17 year-old would be classified as an indecent image of a child. It is illegal to send an indecent image of a child to anyone, even if they are your partner and are also under the age of 18.

4. WHAT HAPPENS IF YOU HAVE A NUDE IMAGE OF AN UNDER 18 ON YOUR PHONE?

You can get into serious trouble if you have a nude image of an under 18 on your phone as this is classed as an indecent image of a child. If an indecent image of a child has been sent to you, delete it immediately.

5. IS IT OKAY IF I TAKE A NAKED PICTURE OF MYSELF IF I AM UNDER 18 AND NOT SEND IT TO ANYONE?

The law states that it is illegal to produce, possess or distribute (make, have or send) an indecent image of a child. So, if you take a naked picture of yourself and keep it on your phone you have still produced an indecent image of a child, even though that child is yourself. It is also important to remember who your phone contract is registered to. If your phone contract is registered to your parent or guardian, technically this means that the phone is theirs. Therefore, if you take a naked picture of yourself using their phone the police would view it as them processing an indecent image of a child. This could lead to serious consequences.

6. CAN YOU GO TO PRISON IF YOU HAVE A NUDE PICTURE ON YOUR PHONE?

Processing an indecent image of a child on your phone is a serious criminal offence. Adults who commit this crime can be sentenced up to nine years' imprisonment (Gov.uk, 2015).

7. WHAT SHOULD I DO IF I RECEIVE A NAKED PICTURE?

If you are sent an indecent image of a child, delete it immediately. Do not show it to anyone or forward it on to someone else as this is classed as distributing an indecent image of a child and is a serious crime. Tell an adult you trust as they can support you.

8. WHAT SHOULD I DO IF A NUDE PICTURE OF ME HAS BEEN SHARED AROUND?

If you have sent a naked picture of yourself to someone and it has been shared with others, this can be very distressing. You may be feeling very upset, but it is important to remember that some adults have been specially trained to help you in situations like this. If the picture is being shared at school tell a teacher you trust or your school's well-being/safeguarding teacher. You will not be in trouble and the teacher will not ask to see the image. If the image has been shared online or on social media, there are ways to contact the site administrators who can remove the image. If it is an indecent image of a child, websites and social media platforms are required by law to remove it as quickly as possible. Always talk to a trusted adult as soon as possible; do not wait and try to deal with the issue on your own.

9. WHAT SHOULD I DO IF SOMEONE IS PRESSURING ME TO SEND A NUDE PICTURE?

It is important to remember that pressuring someone to send a nude picture if they are under 18 is illegal and can have serious legal consequences. If someone is pressuring you to send a nude online, you can block and report that person.

SOURCES OF FURTHER INFORMATION

Brook – www.brook.org.uk

Childline – www.childline.org.uk – this website has a useful section on sexting and online bullying. It also tells you how to block and report sexting on specific social media platforms such as Snapchat, Instagram and Twitter.

CEOP – www.ceop.police.uk

Internet Matters – www.internetmatters.org

Internet Watch Foundation – www.iwf.org.uk

ThinkuKnow – www.thinkuknow.co.uk

✚ CHAPTER 13
CONSENT AND SEXUAL HARASSMENT

QUESTIONS ASKED IN THIS CHAPTER

1. *What is sexual consent?*
2. *Can you give sexual consent when you are drunk or high?*
3. *Can you give sexual consent when you are under 16?*
4. *What is the age of consent in the UK?*
5. *Do you have to give sexual consent in a long-term relationship?*
6. *Do you have to give sexual consent when you are married?*
7. *Can you change your mind once you have given sexual consent?*
8. *What is rape?*
9. *What is the difference between rape and sexual assault by penetration?*
10. *If I have been raped or sexually assaulted, do I have to report it to the police?*
11. *How do I report rape or sexual assault to the police?*
12. *Do men experience sexual assault?*
13. *Can women rape other women?*
14. *What is sexual harassment?*
15. *What are the different types of sexual harassment?*
16. *What is upskirting?*
17. *What is stealthing?*

TEACHER GUIDANCE

Consent does not have to be a controversial issue within the classroom. In order to build the foundations of a good understanding of consent, teachers should start by exploring consent in non-sexual situations with pupils. Specifically, use examples of when we consent in everyday life, for example, when we consent to medical treatment or to have our photograph taken. Teachers should then progress to talking about non-sexual consent in relationships, for example, asking consent before you hug or touch someone. This helps pupils to understand personal boundaries not just within romantic/sexual relationships but also within friendships and between people they interact with in the wider world.

Consent is not just the absence of a no but an enthusiastic yes. It is your role as the educator to make pupils understand the importance of non-verbal consent and body language as well as vocal consent. Pupils should know the physical signs of someone not consenting in a sexual situation such as pulling away during intimate touching or similarly freezing and not actively taking part in sexual interaction. Pupils should understand that these actions indicate a lack of consent. In a wider context, a thorough and effective education around consent allows pupils to understand body language and emotions better.

QUESTIONS

1. WHAT IS SEXUAL CONSENT?

Sexual consent is the agreement between people to engage in a sexual activity. It is vital that there is sexual consent given before any sexual activity takes place. If no consent is given and sexual activity happens, this is non-consensual sex and in some cases rape.

2. CAN YOU GIVE SEXUAL CONSENT WHEN YOU ARE DRUNK OR HIGH?

In the UK, once you have had a drop of alcohol or had any amount of illegal drugs, you lose the legal right to consent to sex (not the physical or verbal ability). If a person who is sober has sex with someone who has drugs or alcohol in their body this is classed in law as rape.

NOTE FOR TEACHERS

To us as adults this may sound a bit shocking. In our daily lives many people will go out and have a drink with a meal or on a date and then engage in sexual activity later that day. While this is true, it is important to remember this law in the context it is being taught. It may be worth pointing out to pupils that due to this law, if you are at a party or social gathering where you have consumed drugs or alcohol, it is probably a good idea to not have sex, as it could be something people regret later. Everyone has different levels of tolerance to alcohol and drugs. One person may drink half a glass of wine and be perfectly coherent while another person may react badly to the same amount of wine and be paralytic on the floor. As a blanket rule to protect everyone the law states that once anyone has any drugs or alcohol in their system, they legally lose the ability to consent to sex.

3. CAN YOU GIVE SEXUAL CONSENT WHEN YOU ARE UNDER 16?

In the UK you are deemed to have the legal capacity (understanding) to consent to sexual activity from the age of 13. Anyone under the age of 12 is deemed not to have the legal capacity to consent to sex and therefore if anyone 13 and over has sex with someone 12 and under, this is automatically classed as rape. If two young people between 13 and 15 are having consensual sex this is not classed as rape but illegal sex.

4. WHAT IS THE AGE OF CONSENT IN THE UK?

The age of consent in the UK is 16 for everyone regardless of their sexuality or gender.

5. DO YOU HAVE TO GIVE SEXUAL CONSENT IN A LONG-TERM RELATIONSHIP?

Yes. Even if you are in a long-term relationship and have had sex with your partner before, consent should be both given and received before any sexual activity happens.

6. DO YOU HAVE TO GIVE SEXUAL CONSENT WHEN YOU ARE MARRIED?

Yes. Just because you are married does not mean you need to have sex with someone whenever they want to. Consent should be given before any sexual activity even if you are married.

7. CAN YOU CHANGE YOUR MIND ONCE YOU HAVE GIVEN SEXUAL CONSENT?

Yes: consent can be given and taken away whenever you want. If you consent to sexual activity but then decide during the sexual activity that you want to stop, you can change your mind and retract your consent. If you change your mind and want to stop having sex, it is important you communicate this to your partner. Do not think you have to carry on having sex if you do not want to, or if you feel uncomfortable just because you have already consented. Your partner should respect you and stop the sexual activity if you want to stop. If your partner carries on with the sexual activity then this is classed as non-consensual sex and in some cases rape.

8. WHAT IS RAPE?

Rape is when a person intentionally penetrates another person's vagina, anus or mouth with a penis, without the other person's consent. Both men and women can be victims of rape. Rape is a serious crime and can carry up to 15 years' imprisonment.

9. WHAT IS THE DIFFERENCE BETWEEN RAPE AND SEXUAL ASSAULT BY PENETRATION?

Rape is when a male intentionally penetrates another person's vagina, anus or mouth with a penis without the other person's consent. Sexual assault by penetration is when a person penetrates another person's vagina or anus with any part of the body other than a penis, or by using an object, without the person's consent (Metropolitan Police Rape and Sexual Assault, 2020). Rape and sexual assault are very serious crimes that can be punished by up to 15 years' imprisonment.

10. IF I HAVE BEEN RAPED OR SEXUALLY ASSAULTED, DO I HAVE TO REPORT IT TO THE POLICE?

If you have been raped or sexually assaulted, there is no legal obligation to report it to the police. It is entirely your choice whether you report it or not. Some people choose not to report rape or sexual assault to the police as they feel they just want to move on and forget about the crime. Other people feel that sometimes they have waited too long to report rape and sexual assault to the police. You can report rape or sexual assault any time after the crime takes place: it will still be taken seriously. No one should ever force you to report rape or sexual assault to the police.

You do not have to report rape or sexual assault to the police in order to get support and advice from charities. See the 'Sources of further information' section at the end of the chapter for charities that can support victims of rape and sexual assault.

11. HOW DO I REPORT RAPE OR SEXUAL ASSAULT TO THE POLICE?

If you have been a victim of rape or sexual assault and have decided to report it to the police, there are several ways you can do this.

+ You can call 101 and report the crime. 101 can also offer you advice on reporting and organisations that can help you.

+ You can use your local police authority's online reporting service. This can be particularly helpful if you are uncomfortable talking to people on the phone or in person.

+ You can visit your local police station and report the crime in person.

+ You can report the crime anonymously through the Crimestoppers website: https://crimestoppers-uk.org

12. DO MEN EXPERIENCE SEXUAL ASSAULT?

Yes, men can experience sexual assault and rape. However, men are less likely to report sexual assault or rape to the police.

13. CAN WOMEN RAPE OTHER WOMEN?

A woman can commit sexual assault on another woman. However, by law rape can only be committed by people with penises.

14. WHAT IS SEXUAL HARASSMENT?

Sexual harassment is the name for any unwanted sexual behaviour that makes you feel distressed or scared. Occasionally, you may experience behaviour from someone that makes you feel uncomfortable, but you are not sure if it is sexual harassment. Regardless of whether you know for sure, you should not feel afraid to speak to someone you trust about your experience if it distressed you.

15. WHAT ARE THE DIFFERENT TYPES OF SEXUAL HARASSMENT?

Sexual harassment can take many different forms and these can include:

+ touching someone without their consent in a sexual way;

+ telling a sexual joke to someone who does not want to hear it;

+ catcalling or wolf whistling someone;

+ making a sexual comment at someone;

+ sending someone graphic or sexual images or videos when they do not want them/was not expecting them;

+ upskirting.

16. WHAT IS UPSKIRTING

Upskirting is when you take a picture beneath someone's skirt or dress without their consent. Upskirting is a serious form of sexual harassment and is illegal in the UK.

17. WHAT IS STEALTHING?

Stealthing is when two partners consent to have sex with a condom and then during sexual activity the male removes the condom without their partner's knowledge. Stealthing is classed as a form of rape and there are serious legal consequences to those who do it.

SOURCES OF FURTHER INFORMATION

Brook – www.brook.org.uk

Disrespect Nobody – www.disrespectnobody.co.uk

Love is Respect – www.loveisrespect.org

Rape Crisis – www.rapecrisis.org.uk

Women's Aid – www.womensaid.org.uk

✚ CHAPTER 14
FEMALE GENITAL MUTILATION

QUESTIONS ASKED IN THIS CHAPTER

1. *What is FGM?*

2. *Where does FGM happen?*

3. *How many girls have had FGM performed on them?*

4. *What are the different types of FGM?*

5. *Is FGM illegal?*

6. *What are the short-term effects of FGM?*

7. *What are the long-term effects of FGM?*

8. *Why does FGM happen?*

9. *What should I do if someone I know is about to have FGM done to them?*

TEACHER GUIDANCE

It is important to not exclude any pupils from learning about female genital mutilation (FGM). While FGM is an issue that affects people with vaginas, it should not just be a considered 'girls' issue'. FGM is a human rights issue. The majority of pupils who are at risk of FGM will be mostly at risk during primary school as FGM is usually done before a girl reaches secondary school. However, you should still be aware as a secondary school teacher of pupils that may be at risk of FGM. If you have any concerns you must report it to your school's safeguarding officer as soon as possible.

It is important to understand that you may have pupils in your class who know someone who has had FGM done to them or has experienced FGM themselves. Due to this, a lesson on FGM can be very distressing for some pupils. Make your classroom a safe and open space by allowing any pupil who wants to leave the lesson due to feeling distressed to leave the classroom for a break or the entire lesson.

QUESTIONS

1. WHAT IS FGM?

FGM is a non-medical procedure where some or all of the external parts of a woman's genitals are removed. FGM can be very harmful, causing both short-term and long-term problems and has no health benefits.

2. WHERE DOES FGM HAPPEN?

FGM happens in over 30 different countries all over the world. It is most common in Africa, the Middle East and Asia.

3. HOW MANY GIRLS HAVE HAD FGM PERFORMED ON THEM?

It is estimated that more than 200 million girls and women across the world have had FGM performed on them (WHO, 2020).

4. WHAT ARE THE DIFFERENT TYPES OF FGM?

There are four known types of FGM that take place all over the world.

Type 1: This is where some or all of the clitoris, clitoral glands and clitoral hood are removed.

Type 2: This is where some or all of the clitoral glands, labia minora (the inner folds of the vulva) and the labia majora (the outer folds of skin of the vulva) are removed.

Type 3: This is known as infibulation, which is the narrowing of the vaginal opening through the creation of a covering seal. The seal is formed by cutting and repositioning the labia minora, or labia majora, sometimes through stitching. Type 3 FGM can also include type 1 FGM.

Type 4: This includes any other harmful procedures to the female genitalia for non-medical purposes, for example, pricking, piercing, incising, scraping and cauterizing the genital area (WHO, 2020).

5. IS FGM ILLEGAL?

FGM is illegal in the UK and many other countries around the world. The punishment for FGM in the UK is up to 14 years' imprisonment. It is also illegal to organise for a girl to be taken out of the UK to have FGM done to them.

6. WHAT ARE THE SHORT-TERM EFFECTS OF FGM?

Some possible short-term effects of FGM can include:

+ severe pain;

+ excessive bleeding (haemorrhage);

+ genital tissue swelling;

+ fever;

+ infections, eg tetanus;

+ urinary problems;

+ wound healing problems;

+ injury to surrounding genital tissue;

+ shock;

+ death.

7. WHAT ARE THE LONG-TERM EFFECTS OF FGM?

Some possible long-term effects of FGM can include:

+ urinary problems (painful urination, UTI);

+ vaginal problems including bacterial vaginosis and infections, menstrual pain, retained menstrual blood;

+ sexual problems (pain during intercourse, decreased satisfaction, etc);

+ increased risk of childbirth complications and newborn deaths;

+ need for later surgeries including deinfibulation to reverse the narrowed opening created by type 3;

+ mental health problems such as depression, anxiety, post-traumatic stress disorder, low self esteem.

8. WHY DOES FGM HAPPEN?

There are many different social and cultural reasons why FGM happens. Mostly they are to do with a society or culture's attributes towards women, hygiene and women's sexuality. Girls who undergo FGM are thought to be 'clean' and make her more likely to receive an offer of marriage. FGM is often considered a necessary part of raising a girl, and a way to prepare her for adulthood and marriage. Parents can be bullied or outcast in their community if they do not let their daughters have FGM done to them. FGM is often thought to be linked to religious practices; however, this is a common myth as there is no religion that advocates FGM.

9. WHAT SHOULD I DO IF SOMEONE I KNOW IS ABOUT TO HAVE FGM DONE TO THEM?

If you know a friend or family member whom you think is at risk of FGM, it is important to act fast and tell an adult you trust who can support you. If someone is in immediate danger, contact the police immediately by dialling 999. If you are concerned that someone may be at risk, contact the NSPCC helpline on 0800 028 3550.

SOURCES OF FURTHER INFORMATION

28 Too Many – www.28toomany.org

Desert Flower Foundation – www.desertflowerfoundation.org

End FGM – www.endfgm.eu

The NHS Website – www.nhs.uk

NSPCC – www.nspcc.org.uk

Plan International UK – www.plan-uk.org

✚ CHAPTER 15
SEXUAL PLEASURE

QUESTIONS ASKED IN THIS CHAPTER

1. What is an orgasm?
2. What is a threesome?
3. What is a sex toy?
4. How old do you have to be to buy a sex toy?
5. Sex always hurts me: is there something wrong with me?
6. What is libido?
7. Is it okay to masturbate when you are in a relationship with someone?
8. Straight men do not use sex toys, do they?
9. Is it wrong to enjoy sex?
10. Can you have sex too much?
11. Is it bad if I have sex with a lot of people?
12. Why do some condoms have dots and patterns on them?
13. What are erogenous zones?
14. What is foreplay?

TEACHER GUIDANCE

This final chapter on sexual pleasure may have come as a surprise, as sexual pleasure is not a topic that is mandatory to teach as part of secondary school RSE.

However, it is vital to discuss sexual pleasure with pupils during RSE, as it can offer guidance beyond the biological and enjoyment aspects of the topic; it can also provide a valuable context for healthy sexual relationships. It is important that every pupil understands that they are entitled to their own sexual pleasure. This means that when they do feel ready to engage in sexual activity, they can be aware of issues that may be symptomatic of an unhealthy relationship. It also empowers pupils to speak out when they feel they are not enjoying sexual activity, because they understand that their sexual pleasure should be a mutually positive experience.

When incorporating sexual pleasure teaching into an RSE curriculum, it does not necessarily require a stand-alone lesson. Rather, it can be explored in conjunction with other RSE topics such as relationships, consent, STIs, sex and contraception.

QUESTIONS

1. WHAT IS AN ORGASM?

Orgasms are an intense feeling of sexual pleasure that can occur when you are engaging in sexual activities. People with penises and people with vaginas can experience an orgasm. They can also be experienced through sexual acts with a partner or if you are engaging in solo masturbation. You may have heard the words 'coming' or 'climaxing'; these are slang words for having an orgasm.

2. WHAT IS A THREESOME?

A threesome is a slang word when three people take part in sexual acts together at the same time. It is important to remember that contraception and consent must be talked about when multiple sexual partners are having sex in the same way that it should be discussed when two people are taking part in sexual acts.

114

3. WHAT IS A SEX TOY?

A sex toy is a device that can be used to stimulate your genitals or different sensitive parts of your body like the nipples or inner thigh. There are many different types of sex toys that can be used by people with penises or vaginas. Sex toys can be used when you are on your own to assist with masturbation or sexual partners can use sex toys on each other.

4. HOW OLD DO YOU HAVE TO BE TO BUY A SEX TOY?

There is no legal age limit for buying a sex toy. However, some sex shops do not let under 18s in their shop because other things may also be for sale, for example, pornography.

5. SEX ALWAYS HURTS ME: IS THERE SOMETHING WRONG WITH ME?

Sex is not supposed to be painful. You may have heard that you should expect pain during the first time you have penetrative sex or every now and again, but this is a common misconception. Sex should never be painful. If you are finding sex painful this could be a sign that the sex is too rough/too fast, you are not aroused (turned on) enough or you are not in the right mental head space to be having sex: for example, you could be too stressed and not relaxed enough. Always communicate to your partner that you are finding the sex painful as this could be a sign you need to slow down, use more lubrication or stop having sex.

Some STIs and medical conditions can cause pain during sex and pain/bleeding after sex. A common medical condition that can cause vagina and vulva discomfort and pain is vaginismus. If this is something you are worried about, it is best to make an appointment to see your GP.

6. WHAT IS LIBIDO?

Libido is another name for your sex drive or your level of sexual desire. Men and women can experience libido. Your libido can be influenced by a number of different factors. Stress, certain medication like antidepressants and hormonal changes like the menopause can cause a person's libido to decrease. This means they will not want to have sex often. Puberty, certain foods and different stages of the menstrual cycle can cause a person's libido to increase, which means they may want to have sex more regularly.

7. IS IT OKAY TO MASTURBATE WHEN YOU ARE IN A RELATIONSHIP WITH SOMEONE?

There are many different opinions about whether you should be allowed to masturbate when you are in a relationship with someone. Some partners may find it upsetting and class it as a form of cheating. It is important to remember that masturbating is normal and healthy regardless of whether you are in a relationship with someone or not. If your partner has a problem with you masturbating, try and communicate with them and ask them to explain why they are upset.

8. STRAIGHT MEN DO NOT USE SEX TOYS, DO THEY?

Using sex toys has nothing to do with your sexuality or gender. Everyone can use a sex toy if they want to.

9. IS IT WRONG TO ENJOY SEX?

No. It is very important that you enjoy sex. You should never engage in sexual activities if you do not enjoy it or do not think you will enjoy it. Some people may engage in sexual activities with their partners because they feel it will make their partner happy or because they think this is what is expected. This is wrong and you should never have sex unless you want to.

116

Some people have ideas and beliefs that women should not enjoy sex and that only men should actively enjoy sex. This can lead to bullying and shaming, and to people with vaginas being called 'slut', 'whore' or 'easy'. This is never acceptable.

10. CAN YOU HAVE SEX TOO MUCH?

Some people worry that there are medical side effects to having a lot of sex such as their penis breaking or a person's vagina becoming 'loose and stretched'. These are common myths. As long as you are practising safe sex by using contraception and engaging in sexual activities with consenting partners, there are no medical side effects to having a lot of sex.

11. IS IT BAD IF I HAVE SEX WITH A LOT OF PEOPLE?

You can have sex with as many people as you want so long as you are practising safe sex and using contraception and everyone who is involved with the sexual activity has consented.

12. WHY DO SOME CONDOMS HAVE DOTS AND PATTERNS ON THEM?

Some condoms have dots and patterns on them to increase the amount of pleasure a person feels during penetrative sex (vaginal, anal and oral sex). The patterned condom causes extra friction, which increases the amount of sexual pleasure felt.

13. WHAT ARE EROGENOUS ZONES?

An erogenous zone is an area of the body that has an increased level of sensitivity due to the number of nerve endings in that area. When an erogenous zone is stimulated (touched, stroked, kissed) then this can cause sexual excitement and pleasure. Examples of erogenous zones are lips, neck, breasts, stomach, inner thigh, genitals and anus.

14. WHAT IS FOREPLAY?

Foreplay is a term given to sexual touching, kissing and stroking before the main sexual activity occurs such as vaginal, anal or oral sex. Foreplay increases sexual excitement in people and increases their feeling of arousal (feeling turned on).

SOURCES OF FURTHER INFORMATION

Brook – www.brook.org.uk

Childline – www.childline.org.uk

The Mix – www.themix.org.uk

✚BIBLIOGRAPHY

Barlow, D (2011)
Sexually Transmitted Infections. New York: Oxford University Press.

Department for Education (DfE) (2015)
Sexual Violence and Sexual Harassment between Children in Schools and Colleges. London: DfE.

Everett, S (2014)
Handbook of Contraception and Sexual Health. London: Routledge.

Merlville, C (2015)
Sexual and Reproductive Health at a Glance. Oxford:
John Wiley & Sons.

NSPCC and PSHE Association (2018)
Making Sense of Relationships. London: NSPCC and PSHE Association.

PSHE Association (2015)
Teaching about Consent in PSHE Education at Key Stages 3 and 4.
London: PSHE Association.

✚ REFERENCES

Department for Education (DfE) (2019)
Relationships Education, Relationships and Sex Education (RSE) and Health Education: Statutory Guidance for Governing Bodies, Proprietors, Head Teachers, Principals, Senior Leadership Teams, Teachers. London: DfE.

Gov.uk (2015)
Sexual Offences Guidelines Consultation: Section Six: Indecent Images of a Child. [online] Available at: https://consult.justice.gov.uk/sentencing-council/indecent-images-children/supporting_documents/sexual%20offences_Indecent%20images%20of%20children.pdf (accessed 24 August 2020).

Metropolitan Police (2020)
Rape and sexual assult. [online] Available at: www.met.police.uk/advice/advice-and-information/rsa/rape-and-sexual-assault/what-is-rape-and-sexual-assault (accessed 29 August 2020).

NHS (2020)
Online contraception guide. [online] Available at www.nhs.uk/conditions/contraception (accessed on 24 August 2020).

WHO (2020)
Female Genital Mutilation. [online] Available at: www.who.int/news-room/fact-sheets/detail/female-genital-mutilation (accessed 29 August 2020).

+INDEX